LABOUR OF LOVE

THE
ULTIMATE
GUIDE TO
BEING A
BIRTH
PARTNER

· · · · · · · · · ·

Sallyann Beresford

db

DANDELION BOOKS

ISBN 978-1-8382295-0-4

First edition: November 2020

Illustrations by Darcy Beresford
Cover and interior design and layout by Tessa Avila
Index by Tessa Avila

10 9 8 7 6 5 4 3 2 1

Printed in the UK

This book is dedicated to my mother, Maureen—
the ultimate birth partner.

She gave birth to me at home in 1970, the story of which I listened to many times over the years of my childhood. It left me with an unwavering belief that my own body was made to give birth. She was with me when each one of my four children were born, and knew instinctively what I needed throughout every birth. Her greatest role in life was that of Grandma, and her bond with all her grandchildren incredibly deep. We love her and miss her more than words can say.

Contents

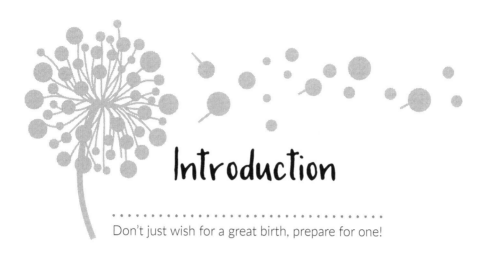

Introduction

Don't just wish for a great birth, prepare for one!

It's happening — you are going to be a birth partner!

How do you feel? Is this your baby, too, or are you a parent, sibling, friend, doula or midwife? Whatever your reasons for picking up this book, I guarantee that it will be the best decision you make in preparation for your role. The right birth partner has the potential to become every woman's secret weapon when it comes to achieving a positive birth. In fact, it is well known and widely documented that a woman who receives continuous support throughout labour—from someone who fully understands what she needs during this time—has a more satisfying experience overall, leading to better outcomes for both her and the baby. Just in case you feel skeptical, because friends and family have been telling you stories of the 'horrors' of childbirth, I will help you recognise why others can, and often do, have such a poor experience. After reading this book, you'll understand that having a great birth isn't about 'luck'.

Whilst there are already plenty of books and useful resources available for pregnant women to learn about their options for birth, until now there has been little to educate birth partners themselves. This book will help change that, as it bridges the gap between traditional antenatal education

1

and what actually happens in a birth room. Each chapter guides you through the process of labour and birth, ensuring that you will know exactly how to put the woman you are supporting at the center of her own experience. I will also help you fully understand why that is so important, and how it leads to a positive birth for all. Throughout, I will share with you all that I have learned about the physiological needs of a labouring woman based on my own experiences of being a professional birth partner for the last 20 years.

> The missing link in most birth preparation is the lack of emphasis placed on the role of the birth partner.

As you read through the book, I guarantee that your confidence will grow. The early chapters will encourage you to open up discussions and give you a wide range of tools to use. This helps you on the day to easily identify what she needs from you or her care providers, and what practical tasks you should be doing for her, based on the list of topics I recommend you cover in the preparation period. The later chapters will ensure that you know exactly how to help her both mentally and physically throughout the birth. By using my PROTECTS tool—outlined fully in Chapter 9—you will know when to feed her body, and when to feed her soul, during the most primal experience of her life. Each woman is unique, and every birth is different, and my aim is to help you understand what to do in any given situation. If, for example, she looks you in the eye and asks for help, she needs to know that she can fully trust you to hear what she is really communicating, because women often vocalise in labour, but do not always want to be rescued. By reading the chapters in this book, you will be able to easily implement the suggestions given, and will soon start to recognise that being a birth partner is about knowing the basic needs of a woman in labour. Once those needs are met, the rest often takes care of itself.

Understanding how the birth process works, and also how the healthcare system works, enables you to feel more confident supporting and advocating if, when or where necessary.

The Reason I Wrote this Book

As a birth doula (professional birth partner), I was typically witnessing wonderful, easy and reasonably quick births with my clients. As an antenatal teacher, however, this wasn't the case. The couples I met appeared to really struggle to cope in the labour room and weren't successfully advocating for themselves in the moment. So I decided to do more preparation work during the course. I changed the format and dedicated an entire session to the role of the birth partner, and the results were incredible. By specifically aiming the content at birth partners, and teaching them the information shared with you throughout this book, I was able to emphasise the importance of the role they played, and it made all the difference. The woman could then relax, making her labour easier overall. She knew that she had someone beside her who was able to recognise what level of support she required, based on the preparation they had done together during the antenatal period.

Whilst every birth is different, and incomparable to another, each and every one should be a positive experience for both the woman and her partner. Learning about hormones, how the baby rotates through the pelvis, and the range of pain relief methods available is a great start, but few antenatal courses, books or classes are able to give you the full picture. You also need to know the role the birth partner plays behind the scenes. That role involves knowing when to step up and be present for her, and when to step back. The latter is important, because many birth partners want to 'fix' birth for a woman, which is not necessary in most cases. By fully understanding her physical and emotional needs, you will gain a level of confidence in the birth process that will help you support her in achieving her dream birth.

The Title of 'Birth Partner'

Throughout the book, you may notice that I always refer to you as 'the birth partner' and the woman as 'the woman you are supporting' so as not to make the assumption that you are her spouse. It is not my intention to offend anyone with the language used. The role of the birth partner is not gender specific, and I want to acknowledge and recognise that there are many women whose life partner is not male, many women who are single, and many people who choose not to identify as women. I also speak about midwives, doctors and other care providers in a way that is not meant to offend such professionals but to alert you to the wide range of situations you may find yourselves in. Women and their birth partners should know that they have the right to be involved in all aspects of the pregnancy and birth process. This book aims to change many of the issues that women are facing within the maternity system, by giving you, her birth partner, the tools to help her feel well supported. Even if for some reason the birth doesn't go to plan, you will have learnt exactly what to do to ensure the birth is a positive one. By remaining in control of all decisions, the woman is much more likely to have an improved perception about her experience, and therefore the postnatal journey will get off to the right start. In writing this book, it is my intention to try to ensure that all women during labour and birth are loved and well cared for, and that their birth partners are confident in their role throughout.

The thoughts, suggestions and opinions offered are not based on any scientific evidence or medical training on my part; they are merely a reflection of my own practice and experience as a doula of over 20 years.

I hope you enjoy the book.

Much love,

Sallyann

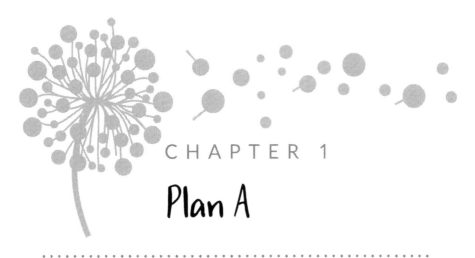

CHAPTER 1

Plan A

Although birth is only one day in the life of a woman, it has an *imprint* on her for the rest of her life.

Justine Gains

The role of the birth partner is reasonably simple, and, to be honest, there is probably less to do than you think. The chapters in this book will help you identify all that you need to know about the physiological needs of a labouring woman, giving you plenty of confidence about what you can do for her during the process. Let's start with helping you know and understand the following:

- What is her 'Plan A'?
- What are the optimal conditions for the type of labour she wants?
- How can you support her in making decisions about her care?

Plan A

'Plan A' is what I call the set of intentions a pregnant woman has decided upon when planning and preparing for her birth. These intentions can include anything—having a home birth, giving birth in a water pool, having an epidural as soon as labour is established or planning a caesarean section (c-section). As her birth partner, your support in helping her identify her ideal birth is important, and no matter what she shares with you, the golden rule is: smile and agree! Whatever she tells you, she needs to know that you will advocate for her, even if it's not a choice that you would personally make.

First Trimester (0-13 weeks)

The majority of women who are pregnant are probably not thinking about the birth in the first trimester. Most women at this stage will still be coming to terms with the fact that they are pregnant, regardless of whether the pregnancy was or wasn't planned. It's an emotional time, and her hormones are busy growing and sustaining a human embryo, which will physically and mentally exhaust her. It might be a long-awaited pregnancy after a difficult time conceiving, or she may have had a miscarriage or two and feel incredibly anxious. Even with a straightforward conception, she is unlikely to be able to focus on anything other than the physical symptoms and sensations she's experiencing. With the end of the pregnancy a very long time away, discussions about her dream birth or 'Plan A' can wait.

The exception is that some women have their birth preferences set in stone before they are even pregnant and are eager to talk about them. I find this is common with women who are expecting their second or subsequent child and who have been through a difficult birth before. A woman in this scenario will often spend months exploring ways to make her next birth different, including possibly hiring a doula or independent midwife. She will usually have set ideas about what she is hoping to achieve, and more importantly, what she is desperate to avoid. Social media groups can become her lifeline; they help her explore and identify which options will enable her to have a better birth experience this time around. In some cases, a woman's options might even include going against medical advice. For example, if she had a previous c-section, she might ask her midwife or doctor about giving birth in a midwife-led unit (MLU) or at home. In contrast, a low-risk woman might want to opt for a c-section. This can lead to some challenging conversations, but she should be able to freely explore and express a wide variety of ideas at this stage. You can expect that your conversations will evolve organically as the pregnancy continues.

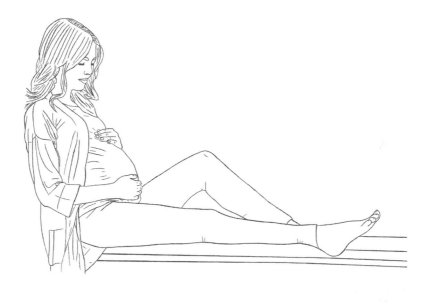

· ·

EMMA'S STORY Emma had a long and difficult first birth, which resulted in a c-section. Her feelings about the experience initially were overlooked with the arrival of the baby, and she was extremely grateful it was over, and that he was here safe and sound. After his first birthday, her antenatal course friends were starting to think about having more children, and it was at this point that she realised that she didn't ever want to go through another birth like her first. She told me that she was really starting to struggle to process her new feelings about what happened to her. I put her in touch with the birth listening service at the hospital, and she was able to go through her notes with a midwife and de-brief her experiences. This really helped her to recognise why she had such a lot of interventions, leading to her eventual c-section. Around the time that her son turned three, she began to research her options and decided she wanted her next baby to be born at home.

She felt confident that this was the best way to avoid interventions, and to have a straightforward, undisturbed experience. She joined an online home birth group and found some like-minded women who helped her to plan her dream birth. Her partner had been unsure about the plan to start with, but the more she shared information about the research she was doing, the more he realised that he needed to support her decision. When she became pregnant, Emma arranged a meeting with the Deputy Head of Midwifery at her local hospital to ensure a personalised care plan was put in place. She spoke about her preferences and how she wanted to be supported to achieve them, even though her previous c-section put her in a 'high-risk' category. At 41 weeks and 5 days, her baby was born at home in a water pool while her four-year-old son slept peacefully upstairs in his bed. It was exactly what she had hoped for and went a long way to heal the wounds left by her previous birth.

Second Trimester (14-27 weeks)

Conversations around birth choices may begin to flow in the second trimester. Don't be worried or alarmed, though, if you get to 20 weeks and beyond and the woman you are supporting is still not ready to think about her options. All discussions can be quite general at this stage anyway, and more serious detailed birth planning sessions can follow, when her decisions will be more relevant—certainly by the third trimester. In the meantime, you can make sure that she is aware of what birth facilities are available to her locally. She can learn about these by speaking to her midwife or doctor, and I also highly recommend she signs up to attend weekly classes like antenatal yoga, where she will be able to meet other pregnant women either online or in person. By listening to the choices other women are making, and hearing about policies and guidelines from the hospitals nearby, she will begin to broaden her knowledge in general. This can help her gain more confidence and recognise within herself what feels right for her and what doesn't. Deciding on the type of birth she wants to achieve may strongly influence the location she chooses (see Chapter 2). For example, if she is interested in a hospital water birth, then she should confirm that it is a valid option at the hospital she has chosen. Some have a reputation for not using their birthing pools very often. To find out, she could ask her midwife, or call the hospital or MLU where she is thinking of having her baby, and ask questions like: 'How many women give birth in water each month, versus how many women give birth in total?' If the water birth numbers are low, then this may indicate a problem, and can help guide her decision. In this scenario, she may even decide to look at switching to another hospital or MLU in her area—one that offers her a greater chance of accessing a birthing pool.

Third trimester (28-40 weeks)

As the third trimester begins, her energy levels will usually start to dip, but her mind will be more than ready to think about the birth ahead. If you haven't already discussed her preferences in detail, then I recommend that you both schedule some birth planning sessions where you can sit down, away from distractions, and truly begin to unpick her thoughts around her Plan A. Invite anyone else who might be with her at the birth to attend these informal meetings, and prioritise them, as they will be very important to her by this stage. I usually suggest that the first one is held around 30–32 weeks of pregnancy, and then another by 35–37 weeks. If you are attending an antenatal course, you could have one session before the course begins, and then another afterwards, as her feelings may change the more she learns about the process of labour and birth. You will then have an easier time during the course identifying and understanding which elements apply to her Plan A.

Birth Planning Sessions

Here are some potential questions to guide your discussion.

1. What are your wishes or preferences for this birth?

2. What are your worries or concerns? Be honest!

3. What do you think might irritate you?

4. What do you want to try or avoid for pain relief?

   - Breathing and relaxation
   - Hypnobirthing
   - Tens machine
   - Water
   - Gas and air
   - Pethidine
   - Epidural

5. What comfort measures or important tasks can I help you with during labour and birth?

   - Touch or massage techniques
   - Hypnobirthing
   - Cold or warm flannels
   - Documentation (photos or videos)
   - Communication with people outside the birthing area

6. Do you understand and have any preferences regarding the following?

   - Monitoring of the baby
   - Vaginal examinations
   - Induction
   - Caesarean section
   - Optimal cord clamping
   - Placenta encapsulation
   - Feeding the baby
   - Skin-to-skin contact
   - Vitamin K

Be Her Rock

As a birth partner, when you talk to a pregnant woman about her 'Plan A', your intention is to encourage her to think about the birth in the most idealised way possible. Remember that nothing discussed at any stage is set in stone, so flexibility is key, but it is important to check in and get a real idea of what she is thinking about. It is also a great way to find out what gaps in knowledge there are between the two of you, so that you can look up information that might affect her decisions during, or just after the birth. If at any stage she feels doubtful about the type of birth she is choosing, just acknowledge her feelings, and perhaps ask her questions without giving your opinion. It is perfectly normal for her to swing between emotions. You do not have to fix anything here; just let her explore and open up as she tries to decide what her Plan A is. As her birth partner, you have an important job! You need to ensure she is aware that she can make decisions about her care alongside her midwife or doctor, rather than having decisions made for her and about her, which can undermine her own belief in her ability to give birth to her baby. She also needs to know that she can trust you and that you won't judge her thoughts about the way she wants to give birth. Always make sure that you:

- Listen to her
- Respect her choices
- Validate her feelings

. . . .

KATIE'S STORY Katie and her partner, Dan, had one child each from previous relationships and were now pregnant with their first child together. Her first birth had not been a positive experience, so when choosing a hospital this time, they had picked one across town that was not the one she had used previously. After attending my antenatal course, she realised that what she really wanted was to avoid an epidural if possible, as she felt that was why she didn't have a positive experience with her first child. She realised that her medicalised birth meant that her movement was incredibly restricted due to the use of equipment needed to support her birth. I suggested avoiding another high-tech obstetric unit where she would be likely to have an experience similar to her previous one. Katie and Dan went to visit another hospital nearby which offered a midwife-led unit, and she switched her care at 38 weeks pregnant. She had a wonderful birth at 41 weeks and 1 day and couldn't believe how different it felt to experience giving birth in a calm and relaxed environment. She shared that the main difference for her was the confidence she felt in her own ability to remain in control of the decisions made about her birth, and she said she felt a huge sense of pride afterwards.

Choice vs Decisions

In theory, women should have choice in all elements of their maternity care, including where they give birth and what happens to them during the process. As part of the Better Births report in 2016, NHS England set up seven maternity choice and personalisation pioneers to test ways of improving choice for women using maternity services, including testing Personal Maternity Care Budgets (PMCBs) as a mechanism for empowering women to take control of decisions about their care. Baroness Julia Cumberlege said in 2018,

> The NHS England choice programme is working to ensure that women are provided with reliable, consistent and objective information on which to make informed decisions, and are supported to understand their options including the risks. This information will support and empower women to make choices that are in line with their preferences and within a clinically appropriate setting.

The Reality

Unfortunately, despite all these important changes going on across the UK, pregnant women and new mums are still indicating that they didn't know they had any choice about what happens to them in labour. Every day I hear women share their stories, saying things like : 'I had to have an induction', or 'I was not allowed a home birth', or 'I wasn't given the option of using water'. They were unaware that they could decline procedures that they had considered routine, such as vaginal examinations, monitoring or induction. They were also never made aware that they had a choice about important events that can really matter in the early moments of birth such as leaving the baby's umbilical cord to stop pulsating after the first minute has passed, or having immediate skin-to-skin contact with their babies during a c-section. Women genuinely tell me that they believed they had no choice at all when it came to medical intervention, even when it prevented them from achieving the birth they had hoped for. Beverley Beech, who was chair of AIMS (the Association for Improvement in Maternity Services) for 40 years, once said at a study day I attended that 'choice is by far the most abused word in maternity services'. For this reason, I cover a wide range of scenarios thoroughly throughout the chapters of this book, including those listed here, so that you will both feel well prepared for all choices that are available to the woman you are supporting. I also recommend that my clients take the focus off the word 'choice' and flip it around to think of everything as 'what she decides'. This makes much more sense to me, and as the birth partner, you should always help her to make well informed decisions. By reclaiming birth and taking back ownership of what happens to her, each woman can begin to understand that she is in the driving seat. It's not about her declining a procedure; it's about her knowing she has the ability to do so if she wishes. All pregnant women should know that they are the ultimate decision-makers when it comes to their birth, and they have the right to choose every element of their care, even if it goes against hospital guidelines. If necessary, an appointment can be made with a community midwife, or a consultant midwife at the hospital, where a personalised care plan can be written and the woman's wishes documented. This will avoid the inevitable 'one size fits all' procedures that come from having guidelines and policies in place that do not suit all women.

> ## No decision about me — without me

Guidelines

Guideline (noun)

A general rule, principle or piece of advice. Synonyms: recommendation, instruction, direction, suggestion

Each hospital works with a set of guidelines that have been decided upon by a multi-disciplinary team. In the UK, these guidelines are usually selected from those of the Royal College of Obstetricians and Gynaecologists (RCOG), The Royal College of Midwives (RCM), the Royal College of Anaesthetists (RCoA), the Royal College of Paediatrics and Child Health (RCPCH) and the National Institute for Health and Care Excellence (NICE). Whilst some of the guidelines are based on evidence and randomised controlled trials (RCT), many are not. Surprisingly, around 40% are decided upon based only on the experience and opinions of the panel who are developing them. You can find out more about these guidelines by visiting the RCOG website, **rcog.org.uk.**

IMPORTANT TO KNOW *If, for any reason, a pregnant woman chooses to decline care based on a particular guideline, her midwife or doctor should acknowledge that the choice is hers to make and then document the discussion in the woman's notes.*

Policy

Policy (noun)

> A course or principle of action adopted or proposed by an organisation
> or individual

The maternity department of every hospital will have an agreed number of rules, or policies. These rules may not be evidence-based and are unlikely to be in the best interests of the woman; they are put in place to limit hospitals' liability. Whilst they are not law, there are some things you cannot change or control at a hospital birth, such as having two birth partners when the policy is one, or using the water pool when you have been told you are not eligible.

Going Against Medical Advice

In some cases, a woman may decide to make a decision about her labour and birth that is not supported by her doctor or midwife. In my experience, any woman who is brave enough to move forward against medical advice, would only do so for a very good reason, and usually only after thorough research. In this instance, it is important that you support her and validate any ideas that she may share with you. If you don't, she will end up feeling disempowered and resentful. During pregnancy, women in this situation are typically on a rollercoaster ride of thoughts and emotions and may struggle to know what to do when pushed into a corner. With the full support of their birth partners, they will always make good decisions, and will never put themselves or their babies at risk. By giving a pregnant woman the space to make decisions about her care, she will inevitably make the right ones.

Personalised Care Plan

You will usually find that when a woman is able to assert herself with a doctor or midwife about her options, the health professional backs down and admits that the woman is correct, and that she absolutely can give birth in the way that she is requesting; health professionals are simply not used to women advocating for themselves, so initially they can often take a strong approach by sticking to the guidelines. In this scenario, once a decision has been made and agreed upon with her care providers, the woman will be given a personalised care plan that is arranged by a senior midwife, and documentation will be written up and put in place behind the scenes to support her wishes. Having you on her side throughout her pregnancy will help her to know that she can trust you to support her during the birth. Plus, in the unlikely event that she has to make the decision to switch from Plan A to Plan B (see Chapter 15), she is less likely to be devastated because she knows she has your unwavering support.

SUSIE'S STORY Susie was pregnant with her first baby, and because she was 40 years old at the start of her pregnancy, she was automatically told that she would have to have an induction at 40 weeks due to hospital guidelines about maternal age. Because she was well and healthy and had only heard horror stories about induction, she decided to do some research, and looked into the evidence available online. She wanted to balance the risks of remaining pregnant past her due date against the risks of having an induction. After a discussion with her partner, Susie felt that she would like to decline the induction until 41 weeks, giving herself an extra chance at going into labour naturally. She spoke to her midwife, and at an appointment with the obstetrician, came up with a personalised care plan that included extra monitoring every other day to check that the baby was doing well. Susie saw her acupuncturist regularly and went into labour naturally two days before her revised induction date.

Resources

Where possible, it is important to make sure that your knowledge about labour and birth supports the information she shares with you about her Plan A. For this reason, I highly recommend, that you both sign up to attend a private antenatal course in your area. You are looking to gain unbiased information that will help you understand the physiological process of giving birth. You might also talk to friends or colleagues and read other books on childbirth. On my website, **birthability.co.uk**, I have provided links to research studies, organisations and blogs that offer factual, evidence-based information. You can also download a variety of free resource material that supports the content of the chapters. The links to this material and more are in the Resources section at the back of the book.

QUICK RECAP

Here are the main things to remember when discussing Plan A.

- **What is her Plan A?** Understand what her dream birth scenario looks like and learn about the optimal conditions that she needs to be able to achieve her Plan A.
- **Birth planning sessions.** Schedule a couple of birth planning sessions together after about 32 weeks, so that you have some dedicated time to talk about her preferences and any other points you want to cover after reading this book.
- **She is the decision maker.** Ensure that the woman recognises herself as the decision maker, and that she understands she should always be the one to say 'yes, please' or 'no, thank you' regarding anything that happens to her.
- **What are the local guidelines?** If it becomes necessary, learn about the hospital guidelines for the NHS trust that she is giving birth under. Regardless of her circumstances, she has the right to discuss and approve the level of care she receives.

CHAPTER 2

Locations

In your local area, there may be several locations to choose from when deciding where the baby can be born. At the booking-in visit, which usually takes place around 10 weeks of pregnancy with a midwife, either in the community or at an initial scan appointment at the hospital, the woman will be offered a series of tests and asked some questions about family history. During that appointment, the midwife may have a discussion with her about where she would like to have the baby. This could be the first time that the woman is made aware that she has decisions to make about her birth. Options should typically include: home birth, midwife-led care in a specialised unit (MLU), or midwife/obstetric care in a hospital. I find that initially, most women will choose to sign up with their nearest hospital, because it's closer and easier. In early pregnancy, this works in the woman's favour, because any appointments that she may be expected to attend are local, involving less travel. As no decisions are set in stone at this stage, she doesn't need to finalise where she would eventually like to give birth until much later in the pregnancy. In my opinion, making a decision about where she gives birth should be fluid and organic, in order for her to get to grips with what feels right. When she is ready to decide, she will need to consider whether the type of birth she is looking to achieve is possible in the location she chooses. Let's say the woman you are supporting would like the option of an epidural. She will need to make sure that she opts to give birth in a main obstetric hospital, or an MLU that is alongside, so that she can transfer if necessary, as an epidural is not available in all settings. What if she wants to avoid induction? In my area, we have five main hospitals to choose from. One hospital books women in for induction at 40 weeks plus 7 days; two at 40 weeks plus 10 days; and two at 40 weeks plus 12 days. You can, however, give birth in an MLU up to 40 weeks plus 14 days. This example shows how important it is to ask around and look at the guidelines of each option in detail, so if the woman you are supporting is keen to avoid induction then it may be best that she books to attend the hospital with the most relaxed policy. This is information that she should be able to access relatively easily herself, or she could enquire through her community midwife. In my last scenario, what if a woman who is pregnant with a subsequent child wants to achieve a VBAC (vaginal birth after caesarean) and avoid interventions? Some hospitals may actively encourage a 'low-risk' style VBAC, enabling the woman to use the water pool in labour, whilst others will not. Instead, they may promote continuous electronic fetal monitoring (EFM) and try to insist on placing a cannula (an intravenous tube) into the back of her hand 'just in case' a problem with her or the baby occurs. Hospitals with this policy may therefore be best avoided. Attending local pregnancy groups or classes and chatting online with other women locally who use the same service will help identify which offers the best options for her. There may also be a local Maternity Voices Partnership (MVP) group or Facebook page where she can read comments of other people's experiences or participate in meet ups that will provide her with the opportunity to connect with other women who gave birth in the same location she is considering.

Low Risk vs High Risk

At that initial booking-in visit with the midwife, each pregnant woman will be assessed to see if she is deemed low or high risk (see Figure 2.1).

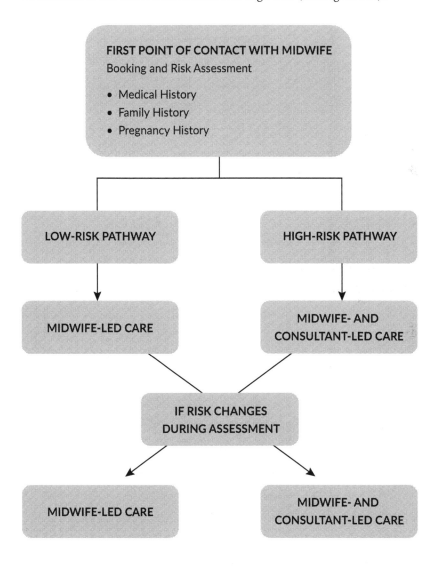

Figure 2.1

The information shared at this visit will be about the woman's previous medical history and any previous pregnancy history. This helps to ensure that she is on the right care pathway. The level of care each woman receives from the outset of her pregnancy will be decided based on this assessment. The woman will be offered straightforward midwife-led care within the normal care pathway if she is low risk, or consultant-led care with midwife appointments alongside for high risk. Each woman will continue to be assessed throughout her pregnancy, and can potentially be switched by her midwife at any time from low risk to high risk or (more rarely) from high to low. It's a shame that the word 'risk' is used at all when assessing pregnant women, as the word signifies danger, a threat, or indeed something unpleasant. Sadly, this is just one of many unfavourable words used within the UK maternity system. As a birth partner, you will need to make sure you know, specifically, how this label might affect her options for the type of birth she is planning. This will help you advocate for her during pregnancy and on the day of the birth so that her Plan A can be achieved.

Low Risk

A woman with a low-risk pregnancy usually has no relevant medical history and no complications or reasons for concern so far. Women who are labelled low risk have an easier time overall because there are no restrictions on where they can give birth, and their pregnancy appointments follow the standard system set out by the NHS low-risk pathway. On the day of the birth, the woman will be encouraged to stay at home for as long as possible in early labour, and when care with a midwife begins, the baby will be monitored intermittently as a matter of routine. This typically involves using an ultrasound device (see Chapter 5) every 15 minutes. Assuming the birth was straightforward, and the mother and baby are well, they can both be sent home after about six hours. If, however, at any point during the pregnancy or labour, a complication with either the woman or the baby develops, it might be recommended that she switches to the high-risk pathway. This can be discussed with a midwife or doctor at the time and should be based on her individual circumstances.

High Risk

In comparison, a woman who is deemed high risk from the outset of pregnancy will receive a lot more attention. This can be for a variety of reasons, but usually because there is a possibility that her or the baby's life can be threatened by complications. She will be expected to attend a larger number of appointments for extra tests, scans and meetings with her consultant, which, due to long waits in the antenatal clinic, can be time consuming. She may be told from the outset what she can expect from the high-risk pathway for her labour and birth, but this will depend on the reasons she is deemed high risk. Any advice at this stage is usually based on hospital guidelines, and may not be personalised at all, so it's important to know that information given can change as the pregnancy progresses, especially if the mother is able to ask questions that relate to her own specific circumstances. An example could be a woman who conceives using IVF (in vitro fertilisation) and is considered to be high risk throughout her pregnancy. If she has no other risk factors, is fit and well, and her pregnancy reaches full term as normal (37 weeks), she should no longer be considered high risk and can request to switch to midwife-led care. This will help her to avoid interventions such as induction, which is typically offered to women who conceived using IVF.

High-Risk Pregnancies During Labour

On the day of the birth, some high-risk women might be encouraged to labour at home naturally for as long as possible; however, if her needs are more complex, she may be advised to arrive at the hospital in early labour for monitoring or medication, begin the labour in hospital with a planned induction, or book in for a caesarean section.

During the labour itself, a high-risk woman might expect to be 'offered' many more interventions—not always beneficial—than low-risk women. An example is the use of continuous electronic fetal monitoring (EFM) of the baby as a matter of routine, despite little to no evidence proving the benefits in any way (see Chapter 5). In fact, research into EFM shows that its use is more likely to lead to increased rates of c-sections and instrumental births, both of which carry risks for mothers. Continuous EFM also makes moving and changing positions difficult in labour, which can impact a woman's coping strategy. It is therefore important that any woman who is deemed high risk, should have a discussion with her doctor during the antenatal period regarding the expectations that will be placed on her during labour. The doctor can then look at her individual needs, and write down her wishes. Documenting at this stage is essential, as the doctors on shift on the day of the birth are likely to be different to the ones she speaks to antenatally. It is not uncommon that a high-risk woman also assumes that she has to have other procedures as standard due to her risk factor, such as an induction. Always remind her that regardless of risk, it is her decision to accept or decline all procedures offered to her.

High-Risk Pregnancies and Postnatal Care

Once the baby is born, depending on the risk factors, the woman and her baby may be expected to stay in hospital for at least 12–24 hours, or in some cases, up to several days. Paediatricians can then continue to monitor the baby's temperature, blood sugar, oxygen levels and heart rate. If the baby is seriously unwell, and has to go to SCBU (special care baby unit) for a prolonged period of time, there is also the potential that the mother will be discharged from hospital before the baby and will need to return each day to visit. This is incredibly unusual for full term babies unless a medical condition was previously diagnosed. In this instance, the level of care required for the baby is most likely to have been discussed in advance. Read more on SCBU in Chapter 16.

A pregnancy might be considered high risk for any of the following reasons.

- An existing medical condition that affected her before the pregnancy
- A medical condition that came about because of the pregnancy
- A medical concern about the baby
- Multiple pregnancy (twins, triplets)
- Previous pregnancy history and/or previous caesarean section
- Maternal weight (BMI)
- Maternal age
- IVF pregnancy
- The position of the baby at full term
- The position of the placenta at full term

Deciding Where to Give Birth

Regardless of the level of risk a woman is labelled as having, she may have more options available to her than she realises. In fact, I have supported many high-risk women in giving birth to their babies in a low-risk setting. Options include the following.

Option One: Home Birth

Many women know from the outset that they would like to give birth at home, and some find themselves drawn to it during the pregnancy. In the end, I don't think that any woman who chooses a home birth makes the decision lightly. Many are likely to receive opposition from partners, colleagues, family and friends with comments such as 'Wow, you are brave' or

'Why would you have a home birth?' In fact, giving birth in the comfort of her own home has numerous physical, emotional and hormonal benefits for the woman, and also has the huge advantage of one-to-one care from the midwives who attend the birth. My favourite benefit of all, however, is that once the baby is born, the mum gets to snuggle up with the baby in her own bed. If you are her spouse or family member, this time is magical, and unlike with a hospital birth, you are not asked to leave when the woman is transferred to the postnatal ward for the night. Instead, you can climb into bed and snuggle up beside mum and baby and have some very meaningful bonding time.

If you are supporting a woman who expresses a desire to have a home birth, and for one reason or another it puts you out of your comfort zone, do not dismiss her idea initially. She needs to explore all of her options and this is a valid one. Many birth partners are not aware that home birth is considered as safe, if not safer than, a hospital birth for most women who remain low risk throughout pregnancy. The Birthplace study, completed in 2010 and published by the University of Oxford in 2011, looked at the data from 60,000 low-risk women, and concluded that giving birth at home was safe, even for first-time mothers, because they were able to avoid major interventions. This is not the same for a woman labelled 'high risk' who would like to give birth at home. In this scenario, there is a balance of risk, regarding her own personal circumstances. If the woman you are supporting would like a home birth after being told that it's not an option for her, then she will need to discuss this with her midwife and arrange for a personalised care plan to be written on her behalf. Her community midwife will be able to help organise this and may even arrange a meeting to discuss the benefits and risks involved. The midwife who facilitates that meeting should acknowledge that the decision is ultimately the woman's to make and deserves support. In my experience, if all options are taken away for reasons that may be based on guidelines and not always relevant to the woman anyway, she can feel incredibly traumatised by any events that happen as a result. Of course, at any time before or during the birth she can change her mind and opt to go to the hospital. I always say to my clients who are considering a home birth that they are better off planning one and changing their mind at any point, rather than realising at the last minute that they would rather have stayed home.

· ·

JILL'S STORY Jill wanted to give birth to her baby at home. During the pregnancy, she developed gestational diabetes (GD). Local guidelines suggested that she should give birth in hospital, and she was encouraged by her midwife to change her home birth plan and have an induction at 40 weeks in case the baby was bigger than average. After some detailed research, Jill felt confident that she would prefer to remain at home and avoid an induction as long as she continued to manage her GD with diet, so she declined the recommendation. She had an appointment with the consultant midwife to discuss and agree on a care plan. Her husband felt a little unsure of the risks and was keen to talk Jill out of the idea of giving birth at home. Eventually, after a broader discussion about the hospital's concerns and the balance of risk between induction and homebirth, he agreed that Jill was making a well-informed decision and felt comforted by the fact that she could transfer into the hospital at any time, if necessary. At 41 weeks, however, Jill attended a hospital appointment with a doctor she had never met before. He told her that she should have an induction and that it was dangerous to continue with her plans to give birth at home. Jill felt she had no choice but to agree and came back the following morning to begin the induction process. She was desperately disappointed by the way that she was pushed to have the induction, and she struggled to relax in the hospital. When her contractions eventually started, about two days later, she was exhausted from lack of sleep and found it hard to cope. In the end her baby showed signs of distress, and Jill gave birth via c-section, which had been her greatest fear. Her son weighed 7lb 10 oz at birth, and she was incredibly disappointed that her baby was of average size and not big at all. Jill was devastated by the way her birth unfolded and felt that if she had been stronger and had declined the recommendation of induction then she would have experienced a beautiful birth at home.

. . . .

Reasons to Transfer from Home to Hospital

Planning a home birth doesn't guarantee that every woman will go on to give birth at home. Some women may decide to change their plans before labour, in early labour, or during established labour. Some will give birth at home, but transfer into hospital after the baby is born. Here are some common reasons to transfer care to the hospital after planning a home birth.

- A condition arises during pregnancy that increases the risk for the woman or baby to remain at home.
- Her waters break with no contractions to follow and infection becomes a concern.
- Midwives find during labour that the baby's heart rate is not responding well to the contractions.
- Midwives at the birth notice significant meconium (baby's first poo, usually seen on a maternity pad after the waters have broken), possibly indicating the baby is in distress.
- The woman chooses to transfer for pain relief.
- The woman simply feels that she would rather be in hospital.
- The woman has heavy blood loss after the birth.
- The placenta has not come away from the uterus despite using oxytocin.
- The woman needs suturing (stitches) in hospital after a significant tear.
- The woman or baby show signs of infection.

I recommend that all my clients research reasons for transfer. This ensures that they will feel well informed about why going into hospital may be advised in any scenario. For instance, in my experience, the presence of meconium (baby's first poo) during a home birth is one of the most common reasons for transfer. However, it's important to understand the difference between significant (fresh) and insignificant (old) meconium. Fresh meconium is thick, black and sticky. If present, it could be an indication that the baby isn't coping with labour, and a sign of distress. Old meconium, which is more of a yellow or green colour, is a sign that the baby opened its bowels before labour began, and is usually not serious. By doing her research in advance, the woman is likely to feel more confident in the event that meconium is present. She will know that she does not have to transfer into the hospital if it is not necessary. She can also ask some useful questions that will support her decision (see Chapter 14). Another common reason for transfer is when the woman herself wants to go. She may be feeling exhausted and is ready to access advanced pain relief options. As the birth partner, you should feel confident that you would know what to do in this instance (see Chapter 3 for information about choosing a safety word).

IMPORTANT TO KNOW   *No matter how much she plans and prepares for a home birth, she may have days in the run up to the birth when she questions her choice. Don't give too many opinions. Simply tell her that you will support whatever she decides. It is perfectly normal for her to swing between thoughts and emotions and absolutely fine for her to change her mind at any point.*

The Birth Bag

If the decision is made to transfer after the midwives have arrived, it will most likely be in an ambulance, depending on the circumstances. As the birth partner, if this is the case, you are not usually able to travel with her. Typically, you are left at home to lock up the house and follow behind in the car with the bags and items for the baby. I suggest for this very reason that all women planning a home birth still pack a 'birth bag' (you will find a handy list of recommended items in the free downloads that accompany this book) so that in the event of a transfer, the birth partner knows where to find everything quickly to grab on the way out the door. The birth bag should contain all the things a woman and baby require, regardless of the chosen place of birth. Ideally you will sit together to pack the bag, so that you are aware of what is inside and understand what comfort measures and snacks are available for you to use (see Chapter 9).

Medical Emergencies

Over 20 years ago, I began running a home birth support group to help other women and their partners understand what was involved in giving birth at home. Couples could meet others who were thinking about a home birth, hear their stories, discuss individual circumstances and have their questions answered by other professionals who joined in with the meetings. At that time, I would often hear concerns about what would happen in the event of an emergency. My answer was always the same: just imagine how much less likely it is that a medical emergency will happen when you are giving birth at home, having removed many of the adrenaline-inducing elements of the hospital in the first place (see Chapter 4). During a home birth, the woman can mobilise easily, and she has one-to-one care from a midwife who is better able to notice warning signs than if she were looking after several women at the same time. I went on to explain that at a hospital birth, even if you were in the room next door to the oper-ating theatre on the labour ward, and a decision was made to perform a caesarean section, it would still take 30–40 minutes to assemble a team, prepare the paperwork, and get the theatre ready for everyone to receive the woman before the procedure began. So if you were at home, and the need to transfer had become obvious due to a problem, assuming you lived within a 30-minute ambulance ride from the hospital, you would still get to the operating theatre in the same time from home as you would if you were already there, as the hospital staff can be preparing for your arrival during the time that you are being transferred.

Independent Midwives

When considering a home birth, many women may not realise that they can hire an independent midwife (IM). These professionals are independent from the NHS, hence the name, but still work to the code that all midwives adhere to. They provide a wonderful service to the clients who can afford them as, like doulas, they charge a fee. For a woman who would like to achieve a birth with minimal fuss and no intervention, they can be of great value, and the relationship that is built between the IM, the woman and her birth partner, and any other children the couple may have is often exceptional. Knowing that the same person you have interviewed and specifically chosen to attend your birth, will come to your home for each antenatal appointment, be on call for you when you are in labour, and will also be there to support you in the early postnatal period, really helps a woman to relax, which can increase her levels of the hormone oxytocin (see Chapter 4) when required. This is especially important for a woman who may be considered high risk by the NHS and has hired an IM because she felt that she was not being supported by her local midwifery team. It is not uncommon for an IM to be asked to support at home: a vaginal twin birth, a breech birth, or a VBAC (vaginal birth after caesarean). Predominantly working in a home birth setting, an IM usually has a high level of experience of observing women give birth with no intervention at all. This is a true physiological birth. This amazing skill stems from the midwives' ability to have the time to develop a trusting relationship with the woman in advance of the birth. You can find more information regarding independent midwives by visiting **imuk.org.uk** or **privatemidwives.com.**

IMPORTANT TO KNOW   *In the event of a transfer to hospital, an IM is unlikely to be able to continue to support the woman in her capacity as a midwife,* *unless they have a special contract with the local hospital. If not, they will still be able to attend, but may step into the role of a doula.*

Option Two: Midwife-Led Unit (MLU)

Many areas across the UK now have the option for women to give birth in a midwife-led unit or birthing center. These are short-stay facilities run by midwives and are proving to be a very popular choice for women who are low-risk and already receiving midwife-led care. There are no doctors available, and therefore minimal medical equipment, which is proven to lower the rates of intervention, and increase the satisfaction of the woman's birth experience overall. MLUs are usually decorated with soft furnishings and home comforts and are often described as being like a spa. The women who choose to give birth in an MLU typically find that the comfort they provide has a positive impact on their hormones, and it helps to be supported by midwives who see birth as being a normal physiological process rather than a medical one.

There are two types of MLU:

1. **An 'alongside' MLU.** This facility has the advantage of being near to or inside a large obstetric unit that also has paediatric care. With options to use water, specially designed equipment, beanbags, mats and other comfort measures, the focus is on mobility as there are usually no beds. Other advantages include multiple birth pools, access to kitchen facilities, and, in many cases, the partner is able to stay with the woman and baby overnight rather than being sent home. Whilst MLUs are predominantly aimed at attracting low-risk women, they will occasionally make an exception for some high-risk women depending on their circumstances. If you are supporting a woman who is high-risk and she would like to consider this option, then my advice would be to encourage her to call and ask to speak to the senior midwife who manages the MLU. She can then arrange a one-to-one meeting, either online or face to face, where they can discuss her own personal circumstances to see if she can be accepted. The criteria for

accepting high-risk women into the MLU varies from hospital to hospital. If she has had a baby before, the midwife can also look at her previous birth notes to establish the reasons why she might be deemed high-risk during this pregnancy, and whether it will affect her chances of having a straight-forward birth. A disadvantage of an alongside MLU is that sometimes, if they are busy on the labour ward, they may close the MLU and move any women in labour across, so they have more midwives on hand. The local community midwife should be able to tell the woman you are supporting if this is common at her chosen MLU and how often it occurs. Alternatively you can encourage her to call the MLU directly and ask them herself. This will help her recognise if this is a valid option for her birth.

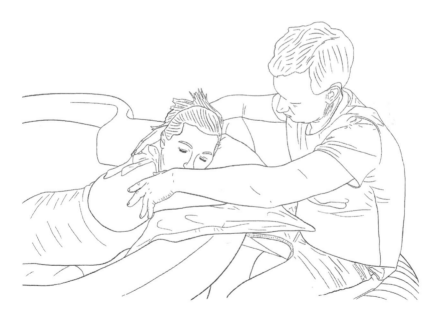

2. A 'standalone' MLU. This is a completely separate facility that is not on the same site as a hospital that provides obstetric or neonatal care. Again, there are no doctors available, and the level of care is similar to what you would expect to receive at a home birth. These units are often staffed by the community team and can be closed at night until a woman is in labour, when they will open up for her just before she arrives. A disadvantage of a standalone MLU is that, just like a home birth, if the decision is made to transfer to hospital in an emergency, it would most likely be in an ambulance.

• •

RAJ'S STORY Raj had a difficult birth with her first child, resulting in a c-section. She was very upset about this, as she'd had a strong desire for a water birth. When she became pregnant with her second child, she told her midwife that she was determined to give birth using the birthing pool, but it was explained to her that the local hospital guidelines didn't 'allow' a woman having a VBAC (vaginal birth after caesarean) to use the water. After hiring me as her doula, Raj contacted a local MLU and asked if we could meet with the manager. At the meeting, they discussed her first birth experience in detail, which was very healing for Raj, and they were also able to ascertain that her current pregnancy was going well. The midwife told Raj that they were willing to accept her onto the unit when the time came and together they wrote a personalised care plan. At 39 weeks and 2 days, Raj had a wonderful water birth and felt that she had finally achieved her dream.

• •

Option Three: Obstetric-Led Hospital Unit

If a woman is deemed high risk and a consultant-led maternity unit/labour ward is considered the safest place for the baby to be born, and the woman is happy with this decision, then it can provide her with an element of certainty when it comes to choosing a place of birth. Many women love this. Modern labour wards are well equipped with everything required for any woman needing additional support, and the level of care provided by obstetricians and anaesthetists is exceptional. If there are any serious risks associated with the woman's health, or if extra support is needed for the baby when it is born, it would be good to know there are these facilities in advance. Make sure you both ask questions about the woman's associated risk, as some information is not always given as standard. You want to determine if there is anything typical about the type of care she might expect to receive during the birth, so it doesn't come as a shock to you both. If you are not her spouse, and are a close family member, friend or doula, then I would recommend you ask the woman if you are able to attend a meeting at the hospital with her to help you to understand what is involved in the type of care she can expect to receive, or be prepared to give her a list of questions that she can ask on your behalf.

If the woman you are supporting is low risk, it's worth knowing that there are a few major disadvantages to her giving birth on an obstetric unit. The main problem is that busy labour wards are, of course, filled with high-risk women often with complex medical needs, and there may only be one midwife looking after several women at a time. In my experience, due to time constraints in large hospitals, interventions may be recommended to individual women on occasion simply to ease the flow throughout the unit. I have personally witnessed this many times, particularly when a shift change was imminent, and a c-section is performed because the theatre is empty and the doctors are trying to pre-empt a disaster where two emergencies come along at once.

That said, if a woman, regardless of her label, would prefer to give birth in a main obstetric unit, as it has access to all the facilities that many women feel more comfortable knowing are there, then this is a valid choice. She may want quick access to pain relief and can relax more knowing that she is in a place that makes her feel safe. In this instance, be sure to talk to her about the higher risk of interventions, and gain her perspective on how she would like things to flow. If she has strong preferences, encourage her to make a list (see birth plans in Chapter 13), then on the day place the list on top of her notes, or hand them to the midwife that is assigned to her upon arrival. You can also ask each new midwife that joins you to read them.

Personalised Care Plans: Making an Appointment

In the event that the woman you are supporting would like to give birth outside of hospital guidelines, and she is told that she is 'not allowed', and is therefore initially unsupported to give birth in a particular way, I recommend you contact the Head of Midwifery, Deputy Head of Midwifery or Consultant Midwife at the hospital where she is booked. Her community midwife will help her to identify who she needs to speak to. Arranging a meeting should be pretty straightforward, and she may ask you to attend with her. You can expect the midwife who facilitates the meeting to help you both understand the risks and benefits of the type of birth the woman is hoping for, and may present you with facts or statements that should be backed up with evidence. Hiring a doula to support you, and contacting organisations like Birthrights and Aims can be incredibly beneficial in this scenario. (See the Resources section at the back of this book.)

Helping Her Decide on a Location

It is important to understand and unpick the depth of a woman's preferences in pregnancy; this makes it easier to support her unconditionally on the day of the birth. Sometimes, she may have deep-seated beliefs that affect her decisions about where she wants the baby to be born, like wanting more monitoring and access to neonatal care, or maybe she is really scared of hospitals. There could be other influences such as medical history, sexual history or a previous pregnancy history that affect her decision about the location of her birth. What is most important is that she researches what is available to her. So many women I meet are completely unaware of the local facilities, and many automatically think they will be 'ruled out' of a particular location, such as home or MLU, just because of a perceived risk factor. Any woman is well within her rights to pick up the phone and ask to speak to the person in charge of an MLU or hospital to enquire about what facilities they have for labour and birth. This way she can be sure that she is going somewhere that ticks all of her boxes, rather than the other way around.

Changing Locations

Sometimes a woman may decide to look into changing her care to another midwife/doctor if the one she is currently assigned to doesn't support her decisions. This is highly recommended, and there will be an alternative medical professional available who shares a philosophy of birth similar to hers. This will make a huge difference to her experience overall, and she can arrange this with a senior midwife at the hospital she attends. If she prefers, she can consider changing to another hospital if she feels this might be more appropriate.

QUICK RECAP

Here are the main things to remember when discussing locations for birth.

- **What locations are available locally?** Be aware of all possible locations for giving birth in the area where she lives, and talk in detail about which will offer the best support for the type of birth she is hoping to achieve.
- **What risk pathway is she on?** Understand the difference between a low-risk and high-risk pathway. If there are any medical concerns for the woman you are supporting, make sure you know if they will have an impact on where she decides to give birth.
- **Remain flexible about location.** Recognise that it is perfectly ok for her to remain flexible about deciding where the baby will be born throughout pregnancy. This means that if she wants to change location at any time, she is perfectly within her rights to do so, and

can contact another hospital to ask them if they will support her in switching her care.

- **Personalised care plan.** If she needs extra support from her midwifery team, she can speak to them about arranging for a personalised care plan. By discussing her own individual circumstances, she can feel confident that they understand what she is hoping to achieve.

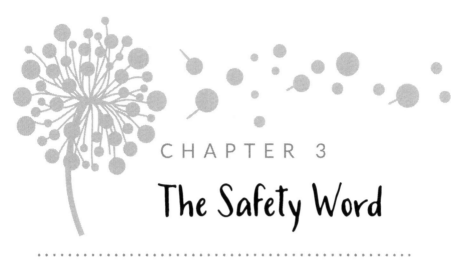

CHAPTER 3

The Safety Word

We have a secret in our culture, and it's not that birth is painful, it's that women are strong.

–Laura Stavoe Harm

A safety word is a word or phrase that the woman chooses before labour and is known by her birth partner to indicate a change in her preferences. As an experienced birth partner, I like to arrive at the birth knowing that the woman I am supporting has access to a safety word if she wants one. It gives the added security of knowing that if she uses the safety word, she wants to change to her alternative plan. It eliminates the guesswork about her wishes and long discussions when labour is intense. It enables you to support her throughout the birth, following her preferences to the letter, whilst confidently knowing that if she is struggling, she has her safety word to fall back on. If at any time she has reached the point where she is sure she cannot continue with her 'Plan A' and wants to access more pain relief, you can confidently step up and get help. The word should be something that she can remember, but doesn't use regularly, so there can be no confusion. She could, of course, just say 'safety word' if she doesn't want to come up with an alternative or she forgets the one she has decided upon in that moment.

Vocalising

It's essential to know that many women will vocalise in labour and share with you that they are finding it tough. It's perfectly normal, and it may carry on throughout. She may have moments where she doubts herself, moments where she has a good cry, and she may have moments where she simply doesn't want to go on. What is important to her is knowing that you have her back, are protecting and supporting her wishes and won't let her fall at the first or even last hurdle. This can happen when a birth partner tries to 'fix' a birth when it doesn't need fixing! What I mean by this is that it's not uncommon for an inexperienced birth partner, particularly if it is her spouse or mother, to struggle when witnessing the woman in distress. They can often, unintentionally, say words that undermine her goal, simply because they want to help her. Occasionally a woman might become annoyed with her partner if she is struggling during a particular phase. It is important not to take anything she says during labour personally, and as I always tell my clients, 'what happens in the birth room stays in the birth room'. As her birth partner, you have a very important role: you have to trust her body as much as, if not more than, she does. You have to believe in her ability to give birth more than she does, and you have to be stronger than she is, so that even if she looks you straight in the eye and says 'I don't want to do this anymore', you can confidently say 'You can, I'm right here, and you are doing great'.

The Marathon Analogy

Let's pretend she has signed up to run a marathon: something she has made a decision she wants to take part in. By signing up, she has made a big commitment, trained well, collected sponsorship money and bought all the gear. She has done a lot of research, and has some set ideas about how she wants the run to go. She has prepared both physically and mentally and has a running buddy who she trains with. As the big day approaches, she starts to have doubts about her ability to finish the race. Even though she

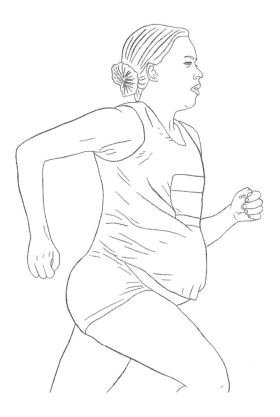

has been sure to surround herself with people that encourage her and help her through, she has last-minute nerves. You tell her she is amazing, and you watch her set off and agree to see her at the finish line. As she runs past you on the way, you see that she is struggling. It's really obvious to you, but even though it is tempting, you don't yell at her to quit and come home—of course you don't! As the race continues, you might notice that she is limping and in pain. Even though you can see she is crying, you also know that she is trying to keep going and wants to finish. You wouldn't shout out to her 'There's no need to be brave! Just stop now and we can go to the pub for some lunch!'—of course you wouldn't! You are more likely to run next to her during the race, encouraging her through that final mile by keeping her company and spurring her on.

For some reason, when it comes to having a baby, many birth partners simply don't know how to help the woman cross the finish line. Vocalising and acknowledging they are struggling are a normal part of the birthing process for most women, so there is no need to say things to pacify the situation. You should simply keep her going—unless she 'safety words' you. You would be amazed at how many times I have heard statements like 'No one will give you a medal for not having pain relief', or 'Shall I get you something to take the pain away?' Whilst I am not suggesting that a woman should avoid pain relief, if it is her intention to try, then her supporters on the sidelines will make all the difference if they can sit quietly, spurring her on only when she needs it. Then, if she does decide to step away from her Plan A, she will be making that decision for herself.

Knowing a safety word is in place will:

- help you feel confident to keep her going within each moment for as long as she wants to.
- reassure her that she can express herself as much as she wants without worrying that you will give up on her.
- help all medical providers to understand that whatever happens, they should stick to her list of preferences unless she uses her safety word (or a medical need arises).

By discussing in advance that you will be encouraging her during the times when she's struggling, she will know that she can vocalise without worrying that you will doubt her ability to cope. To be able to hear a woman tell you she finds it hard, as many times as she wants, and to know that you can never push her too far is essential. You want her to know that she is able to trust you, and that includes getting her help when she asks for it. So at any point, if she uses the safety word, you must stop and get help. You might say 'I hear that you are finding this tough and you have just used your safety word. How would you like me to help?' At this point you can have a discussion about what the next step looks like. This way, you will always be confident that she will never have regrets. She will never feel that you didn't support her, and she will know that she was always the one who had control over her labour and birth.

Statements You Might Hear

I find that, typically, women can have a series of 'wobbles' at different points during labour. Having never performed a vaginal examination, I can't say for sure, but usually I would expect to see a wobble or two around 5–6 cm, and then again around 9–10 cm. During the earlier ones, women will express their fears or doubts in their ability to continue. This is normal, and you should say very little, except soft gentle words to encourage her. For example:

- When she says, 'I can't do this anymore', you say 'You are doing it.'
- When she says, 'I am really struggling with these contractions, they just keep getting worse', you say 'Use your breath—you're doing great.'
- When she says 'I want them to stop', you say, 'I know—let's just get through a few more.'

These earlier bouts of vocalising tend to pass quickly when she hears your confident responses. If she is using gas and air at this time, be aware that she can feel a little out of control, which might make her forget what she is trying to achieve. If she begins to use the gas continuously and for longer than the length of each contraction, then I recommend you offer to hold the handle of the mouthpiece in between. As each one ends, you take hold of the handle, and then encourage her to relax and flop all her muscles between surges. Keep the handle close by, so she knows she can access it easily, anytime she needs to. This break between contractions will help her keep a clear head.

Later wobbles tend to be much more serious! She may be definite that she does not want to carry on with the labour—she tells you she wants help, and she wants it now! At this time, there is every possibility that she could be around 9–10 cm dilated, and that the wobble is brought on by a surge of the hormone adrenaline. This may signify that she is entering transition. I am usually excited when a woman starts to show signs that she is losing her resolve. In this moment, it is important for you to keep your cool and think logically. Feel her lower legs and see if they are cold to the touch, as this can indicate she is almost fully dilated (see Chapter 5).

Using the Safety Word

If she uses the safety word at any point during the labour, then your response should be pretty clear. You say, 'Ok, I'm listening!' You then need to understand exactly what is happening for her. If she has been using gas and air, you might need to ask her to stop for one or two contractions so that it wears off. It is common for a woman using this method of pain relief (see Chapter 12) to be so high that they feel totally out of control and won't realise what they are saying. If possible, you want to avoid this scenario. Once she has regained awareness, you can then have a sensible discussion with her, and she will be able to remember what she is saying. This will help you both to feel confident in any decision she makes at this time. During the conversation, listen to her instincts. Some women will say things like 'It's just not happening' or 'I'm not progressing'. If the woman knows that something is not quite right, it might be that external support is required, and it is appropriate to switch to Plan B at this time. One caveat to keep in mind, however: when a woman is nearing the end of the first stage of labour (see Chapter 5), there is the potential that she may use her safety word because her hormones are doing the talking. She may be experiencing a huge surge of adrenaline (the fight or flight hormone) and she could be letting go of her dream birth prematurely. It is a big step to get out of a pool, transfer from an MLU to labour ward or even from home to hospital. If the safety word is used, regardless of the scenario, and you suspect she may be more dilated than she thinks, then you could ask her if she would like to know how progressed she is before making that final decision. She could speak to her midwife about a vaginal examination

(VE) to see if it provides her with some additional information. Whilst a VE is not something I would normally suggest, as it can be inaccurate (see Chapter 14), I think in this instance the offer is important as it can help the woman remain in control. If she is in transition and almost fully dilated, then she may decide to carry on with Plan A; however, if she is not and she feels she definitely wants to switch to Plan B, then she can move forward with confidence.

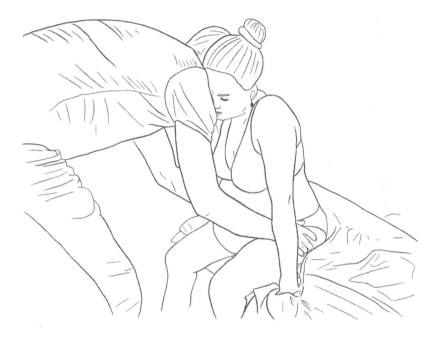

Choosing a Safety Word

This needs to be something that she wouldn't normally say—a word that you will both recognise, but couldn't easily be mistaken. Try not to over-think it. If she can't think of one, or forgets it on the day, then she can just say 'safety word' or 'I'm *#!% safety wording you!' and you will soon understand what she means!

It's incredibly important to have a discussion about this process during the antenatal period, so that you can get a really good idea of her threshold, and what that means. Not her 'pain threshold'; I am talking about her fears and her 'doubting' threshold.

Every woman will approach pregnancy and the birth preparation period differently. Some will be open from the outset and express a wish to try different methods of pain relief, and some will know that they would like to use a water pool or give birth at home. For all these scenarios, a safety word is incredibly useful. It will give you security and bring you peace of mind knowing that you can stick to Plan A and encourage her to keep going even if she looks you in the eye and tells you 'I really can't do this anymore'. You will have the confidence to say how amazing she is and how you are going to be right by her side. You are not going to push her because you are cruel, but because you would not want her to feel like you let her down by not supporting her wishes. Having a tool that protects you both is essential.

Let's look at a couple of examples where you might feel unsure about what to do should a similar scenario arise.

Example 1

Amy had been attending pregnancy yoga classes each week and had decided that she wanted to have a water birth. She bought a hypnobirthing CD and had been listening to it each night during the last weeks of the pregnancy. She had told her birth partner that she wanted to try to avoid all forms of pain relief, and had written on her birth plan that she didn't want to be offered any, but noted she would ask for some if required. After she arrived at the hospital, she requested use of the birth pool. It took a while to be ready, and Amy was starting to vocalise she was struggling, as she was desperate to get in the warm water. The midwife explained it would be a little while yet, and she offered her gas and air, which Amy agreed to. As soon as she started to breathe the gas, she liked it. Very soon afterwards, she was a little 'off her head', and became heavily reliant on using the gas at all times with no break. What should you do?

1. As soon as the midwife suggests gas and air, take her aside and ask her to read or re-read the list of Amy's birth preferences. Quietly and politely point out that Amy doesn't want to be offered anything, including gas and air, and that she has a safety word in place that she will use if she changes her mind. Then carry on supporting Amy through each surge, not mentioning it again, unless Amy brings it up herself.

2. Ask Amy to confirm that she is happy to accept the gas and air, and tell her that you need to hear her use her safety word.

Example 2

Sophie has stated from the outset that she would be open to any form of pain relief in labour. Her preferences are very flexible and she has no fixed ideas about how her birth will go. Labour begins at night and she waits until morning before heading into hospital. When she begins to vocalise, she is very clear and looks at her birth partner with certainty stating that she wants an epidural. She hasn't safety worded yet. What should you do?

1. Ask her outright 'Can I just check—are you going to use your safety word?'

2. Ignore her and encourage her to keep going, even though you know she wants an epidural.

Answer: It's really tricky, but I do believe that you have to gauge which route to choose based on the discussions you have had in the antenatal period. You should know her well enough to decide which option to go with. If in doubt, always choose to move past her comments unless she safety words you, if this is what you have agreed in advance. It would be a real shame to sit opposite someone after the baby is born, and have them tell you that they regretted making a major decision too early in the labour and that they felt they had made a mistake. In my experience, no matter how clear and consistent a woman has been about the flexibility of her preferences, you should still not act until she uses the safety word if she has agreed to put one in place. I have made this mistake before.

IMPORTANT TO KNOW *If she tells you she doesn't like the idea of having a safety word at all, then at any point during labour and birth, no matter what she asks for, you should listen. Or, if it becomes clear that an emergency situation requires an immediate switch to Plan B with her consent, then it can be assumed that the safety word is no longer applicable.*

QUICK RECAP

Here are the main things to remember when discussing the use of a safety word.

- **How a safety word is beneficial.** Talk together about the principles behind the use of a safety word, and how agreeing on one could benefit you both during labour.
- **What is her safety word?** If she is happy to use one, what is her chosen word? Encourage her to think of a meaningful word that she would not typically use on a regular basis.
- **When would she use a safety word?** Talk together about the scenarios where she might use a safety word, and what she thinks her Plan B might look like in that instance.
- **Making decisions.** Recommend that if she uses her safety word whilst she is high on gas and air, that she has a break for one or two contractions before you have a discussion around how to move forward with Plan B. Ask her how she would feel about having a vaginal examination (VE), if using the safety word involved her making a major decision about her birth.

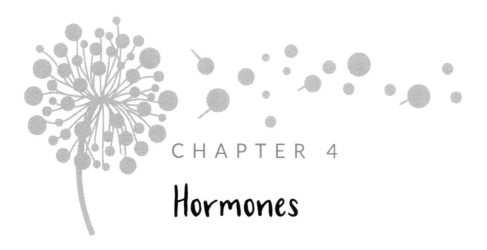

CHAPTER 4

Hormones

One cannot actively help a woman to give birth. The goal is to avoid disturbing her unnecessarily.

–Michel Odent

The key to truly understanding the physiological needs of a labouring woman lies with your knowledge of hormones. If you don't 'get' hormones, you won't 'get' birth! Take your time reading through this information and make sure you know it inside and out, because understanding the role that hormones play in getting a woman into labour and keeping her there is an essential part of being a birth partner. It sets the foundation for all the remaining information that will follow throughout this book. Whilst this chapter begins with a very brief overview of the wide range of hormones released by a pregnant and labouring woman, I believe you only need to focus on the top three, which I will explain in detail.

Hormones are required to:

- **Grow a healthy baby.** As a pregnancy begins, oestrogen and progesterone levels rise, helping the fetus to develop and mature. The hormone relaxin starts to loosen the body in preparation to accommodate the growing baby. Some women may experience pelvic girdle instability as ligaments and the symphysis pubis joint within the pelvis begin to soften.

- **Signal that the baby is ready to be born.** At the end of pregnancy, the baby will outgrow the space in the womb, which causes a stress reaction in the baby and the uterus. A cocktail of hormones is released by both baby and mother, and her body starts to prepare for birth. Progesterone, which has been essential throughout pregnancy to keep the cervix tightly closed and prevent labour, now begins to decrease.

- **Synchronise contractions in the uterus.** As the levels of two of the most important hormones—oxytocin and prostaglandins—rise along with the hormone relaxin, the cervix will start to soften and ripen. Some women will feel contractions at this stage, and some may not. As the woman produces more and more oxytocin, the contractions begin to synchronise, and the cervix starts to open.

- **Produce natural pain relief.** When the body is in pain or stress, beta-endorphins are released to bring the body back to balance, a process called homeostasis. Beta-endorphins are a reward to the body for its hard work. They reduce the effects of stress, and induce feelings of pleasure and euphoria similar to the response a woman would get if she was given an opioid, like morphine. They increase over the duration of the labour and peak after the baby is born, leaving the woman feeling euphoric.

- **Dilate the cervix.** Oxytocin levels continue to rise, causing regular contractions of the womb and abdominal muscles. Oxytocin-induced contractions become stronger and more frequent as progesterone and oestrogen levels fall. The woman may experience more intense surges as the cervix opens and thins out around the baby's head.

- **Energise the mother so she can push out her baby.** At the end of the dilation process, the mother is filled with a surge of adrenaline: the 'fight or flight' hormone. It is responsible for providing a labouring woman with all the energy she needs to push her baby into the world. She becomes wide-eyed and alert, and her blood is pumping to her heart and limbs. She may not realise in that moment that she has the strength to push, but if she trusts her body, it will do everything for her.

- **Complete the bonding process.** Once the baby has been born, the woman needs another surge of oxytocin to help her uterus contract. This is produced alongside prolactin as the mother holds her newborn baby skin-to-skin, and gazes into his or her eyes. Whilst not all mothers feel an instant bond with their babies, the presence of high levels of oxytocin and prolactin are fundamental in helping the process along.

- **Prepare the body to feed the baby.** After the placenta has separated from the uterine wall, levels of oestrogen and progesterone drop even further, enabling the woman to produce colostrum: a high-density milk ideal for newborns. As the baby feeds, high levels of oxytocin and prolactin are released from the mother's pituitary gland, stimulating more milk production and bonding.

> Without the right hormones, there will be no labour!

The Three Main Hormones

Whilst all of these hormones are vital in their own way, I want to focus on just three in particular that have the biggest impact on the physiology of labour and birth.

1. Prostaglandins
2. Oxytocin
3. Adrenaline

Prostaglandins

Prostaglandins are essential for the early stages of labour. The cervix must change and go through what is described by medical textbooks as 'cervical ripening'. The softening and ripening process will help the cervix to shorten and thin out so that it can then begin to open and move out of the way for the baby. There is a lot of physiological work going on behind the scenes that needs to be acknowledged, especially if the woman is aware that labour has started, and she feels that progress is slow. As her oxytocin levels rise, she will begin to produce contractions. This part of labour, known as the 'latent phase', is the period of time when contractions can vary in frequency and length (see Chapter 5). The longer the latent phase, the more exhausting labour is for the woman. This is a time for sleeping or resting as much as possible. She should eat delicious and nutritious foods, whilst drinking plenty of water to hydrate her body. Regular trips to the toilet are recommended, as she should empty her bladder regularly, ensuring the baby has as much room as possible to move down. Advice given by her midwife at this stage might be to 'take a couple of paracetamol and have a bath', but I recommend that she avoid both if possible. Many of the over-the-counter pain relief remedies that she may have at home can actually prohibit the production of prostaglandins, leading to a longer labour overall. If she does want to take a bath, ask her to lie on her side, and not on her back. Staying off her back—wherever she wants to rest—will ideally keep the baby in an optimal position, or help it to turn with each contraction. The start of labour is a very delicate time, and it is important to avoid chasing the contractions, which will exhaust her. Rest, rest and more rest is all that is needed at this stage.

Oxytocin

Oxytocin is the 'Big Cheese' of birthing hormones. It is required to produce contractions in the first and third stages of labour. Oxytocin has a few nicknames, including 'hormone of love', 'cuddle chemical' and 'the hug hormone', because in order to secrete it, a person needs to feel loved and safe. As well as during labour, a woman is likely to produce an abundance of oxytocin when she is surrounded by her friends or family, eating a delicious meal, playing with her kids or her pet, and during sexual arousal and orgasm. At all of these times she is typically relaxed and enjoying the moment, rather than feeling stressed or anxious.

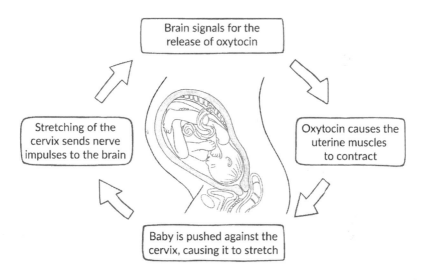

Figure 4.1 The production of oxytocin is controlled by a positive feedback mechanism. It is released when a trigger occurs, and as long as the body continues to receive the trigger, it will create more and more.

Oxytocin is controlled by a loop called a feedback mechanism (see Figure 4.1), and as labour begins, it is initially triggered by the baby. In order for it to continue to be produced, the woman needs to experience many or all of the optimal conditions that oxytocin requires. The more she produces, the more the body will make. Without high levels of oxytocin, there will be no contractions and therefore no dilation. This means that if the woman's oxytocin levels dip, progress will slow, leading to a longer and therefore often more difficult labour. She may become tired and disheartened, and if the loop stops and the body does not continue to produce oxytocin at all, interventions may be recommended, including a synthetic version of the hormone called Syntocinon.

Oxytocin is a hormone that is produced in abundance when the woman feels safe, loved, warm, comfortable, and is in a quiet, dark and private environment. In addition to positive affirmations and words of gentle encouragement, here are some practical items to help a woman produce oxytocin.

- **Comfortable pillows that smell like home.** I recommend trying to fit two pillows into one pillow case to make it more dense and therefore more comfortable for her to lean on and relax into.
- **An eye mask.** If the room is too bright, she will produce less oxytocin and labour can take longer. Many women will automatically close their eyes, but light can filter through her eyelids and still affect her, so consider closing the curtains or blinds. If she wants to take a string of battery lights to her birth, make sure they are warm white, not bright white, as the blue light emitted from bright white lights can overstimulate the brain.
- **Relaxing background music.** Many women prepare a playlist in advance of the birth. I recommend she has headphones in her bag, in case the environment is noisy.
- **Soft blankets.** These are useful to cover her up and keep her feeling warm, which can also offer her a sense of privacy.
- **Pleasant scents.** Essential oils like lavender can help her feel calm and relaxed.

Adrenaline

Adrenaline is a hormone that is produced in abundance when a labouring woman is easily distracted by: fear and doubt, overanalysing of her progress, a lack of privacy, discomfort, too much sound or light, or too many questions. Whilst adrenaline is required in abundance during the second stage of labour, if it is introduced into the body too early, it will counteract oxytocin production, causing labour to slow down or stop. If the woman comes out of her 'oxytocic bubble' during the first stage, it is most likely because she is releasing adrenaline, and her feedback mechanism loop will be broken, leading to a longer labour. It is therefore important to recognise that adrenaline is a serious enemy to the production of oxytocin, and should be avoided as much as possible whilst a woman is dilating. As her birth partner, it is your job to know what can cause an adrenaline spike to occur, and help to protect her oxytocin where possible.

· ·

NICOLA'S STORY Nicola was pregnant with her first baby. She suffered from anxiety and was worried about how she would cope in labour. We discussed all her options, and she decided that she would like to give birth in her local 'alongside' MLU, knowing that she could transfer to the hospital labour ward if necessary. Nicola went into labour at 40 weeks and 5 days, and during her time at home, she struggled to relax. She was in what I would describe as 'high alert' mode and was becoming very tired. A community midwife was able to come to her house and assess progress on two occasions. Unfortunately, during both examinations, which were eight hours apart, Nicola remained just one cm dilated, which was extremely disappointing for her. She coped really well with the contractions, but as hard as I tried, I couldn't get her to relax. As time went on, I recognised that she needed to let go of the thoughts that were holding her back, as she constantly analysed her labour. We agreed with the midwife that even though she was still in the very early stages, she would benefit from going to the MLU, having some pethidine (see Chapter 12) and relaxing in the pool. This worked really well for her and when she was checked again four hours later, she had dilated to six cm. The pethidine enabled Nicola to switch off her anxious thoughts, and in doing so, it reduced her adrenaline levels so that her oxytocin could pick up again and her cervix began to dilate.

. . . .

Helping a Woman with Too Much Adrenaline

In my experience, a woman who has high levels of adrenaline tends to appear as if she is trying very hard to relax, but in reality has one eye half open all the time, is hyper-alert, and unable to switch off. She may be trying to control the labour and bring it on before it is ready or she may be overanalysing what she is experiencing. Even telling her to relax, in itself, can produce more adrenaline in this scenario.

It is important to eliminate any excitement, and to gently encourage her to hunker down and rest. I highly recommend she lies on her left side, or perhaps gets into a comfortable position leaning forward over a pile of cushions or a ball, helping her to conserve all her energy for later. You will be able to see if it is working, because as the hormones build, contractions will become longer, stronger and more frequent, and if they don't, then something is stopping them. Getting her comfortable is important to help her try and switch off from overthinking (see Chapter 8 for ideas on positions). Ideally, you want the room she is in as dark as possible, and you want to stay out of her line of vision and avoid conversation. At this stage, if she is willing to be left alone, but confident to know that you are close by, stay out of the room as much as you can. I find that a woman who feels too observed will begin to feel under huge pressure to perform. If you can see that she is nervous, anxious or excited and is doing a lot of active thinking and talking, then she will need you to encourage her to let go of that level of control (see Chapter 10).

JESS'S STORY Jess was expecting her second baby and was given a date for an induction at 42 weeks. She felt pretty stressed out about it, but went into labour at 3 AM the morning before. She arrived at the MLU at about 8 AM, and was shown into a room with a pool, which was in the process of being filled. The midwife told her that if she wasn't in established labour, she would still be expected to attend her appointment with the doctor for the induction. This really upset her, and it's no surprise that during the time the midwife was in the room, Jess did not have a single contraction. I arrived shortly afterwards, and she was contracting beautifully, but sure enough, when the midwife came back into the room it all stopped again. The midwife became quite adamant that Jess could not possibly be in labour, stating she could only go by what she was seeing, despite our reassurances that she was contracting beautifully. I recommended that we swap to a different midwife, and while all that was being organised, I was able to get her into the pool. By the time the new midwife came into the room, about 20 minutes later, Jess was contracting consistently and showing signs that she was ready to push. The new midwife was shocked to discover this, as she had been informed that Jess was still in the early stages. She rushed around trying to get everything ready as the baby was born into the water. In this situation, Jess's contractions were literally knocked out by the presence of someone who made her feel unsafe!

Parasympathetic and Sympathetic Nervous Systems

When a woman is producing high levels of oxytocin, her parasympathetic nervous system is in flow. Otherwise known as 'rest and digest', this state keeps her heart rate low, and blood flows away from her muscles towards her digestive and reproductive organs—in particular her uterus.

It also causes her to feel quite sleepy, easing her into that oxytocic bubble. In comparison, when she is producing high levels of adrenaline, her sympathetic nervous system is in charge—otherwise known as 'fight or flight'. Her body is prepared to run, so she is wide-eyed, and all her blood is pumping to her heart and limbs. These two divisions serve the same organs, but create opposite effects in the body. They either excite the body's functions or subdue them. One amps you up and prepares you for activity while the other talks you down, undoing what the other did. Our ability to enter fight or flight when we are facing life or death is what has kept our species alive; if a sabre-toothed tiger came around the corner, we would definitely want all our energy to go to our brain, heart and muscles, or we would not have the ability to run fast. Unfortunately, in modern times, our stress responses are triggered far too frequently as a reaction to our physical or mental equilibrium. This response can be caused by looming deadlines, financial issues, an argument with a loved one or feelings of being overwhelmed. It is fair to say that many of us live in an almost constant state of stress, with the body barely ever getting a break. As a birth partner, you will need to understand how easily 'stressed out' the woman you are supporting can get. Talk to her about her fears and beliefs about giving birth, and see if you can get to the bottom of the type of things that might hold back her relaxation response.

Sympathetic Response

During the early stages of labour, even a small stressor can signal a problem to the woman's body, and she will begin to produce adrenaline. As the uterus is not required or essential for the body to survive in a threatening situation, blood is therefore pumped away from it. This causes arteries going to the uterus to tense and constrict, restricting the flow of blood and oxygen. It's easy to see why labour might be slow in this case (see Figure 4.2).

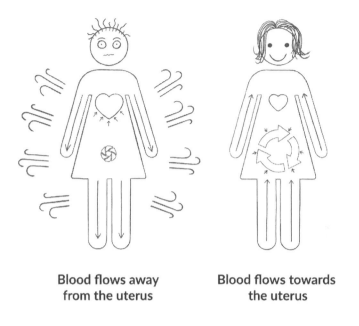

Blood flows away
from the uterus

Blood flows towards
the uterus

Figure 4.2 Sympathetic and parasympathetic nervous system

Parasympathetic Response

When a woman has high levels of oxytocin, she is in the parasympathetic state of 'rest and digest'. She is in a deep labour zone that enables her body to work with no input from her brain. It is such a deep effective state, that the more she relaxes, the more oxytocin is produced. This in turn brings on more contractions. In a parasympathetic state, where she is maintaining a calm and relaxed environment, a woman dilates faster and feels less pain. By learning about the power of the parasympathetic nervous system, you can recognise it as one of the key players to success for the birth you attend. With the additional tool of hypnobirthing (see Chapter 11), the physiological effects of the parasympathetic response can enable the woman's body to eradicate the adrenaline, (apart from those moments when adrenaline is required for the birth process), leading to a shorter and more efficient birth overall.

Thinkers and Planners

Thinkers and planners tend to be very organised women, and whilst these are fortunate qualities to have, they don't work well at a birth. These are the minds that struggle to switch off the most. If you suspect the woman you are supporting is likely to need extra help at her birth, it is important to get her to understand the differences between the sympathetic and parasympathetic nervous systems. Once she is able to recognise the need to let go of all that she has learned in her pregnancy, she will find it easier to trust her body. She can feel confident that her subconscious mind has stored everything safely, and she will be able to recall information if she needs to. You can also recall it for her because, as her birth partner, you will by this point know everything that matters to her. In the event that she cannot relax and switch off, and the labour becomes long and she is tired, you could consider speaking to her about using some gas and air (see more about pain relief in Chapter 12). Perhaps if still in the early stages she can think about pethidine. In extreme cases, this can work really well, because she is able to relax and switch off her thoughts perhaps for the first time that day. By talking to her in advance about how she would feel in this kind of scenario, you can ensure that she understands how important it is for her to keep adrenaline at bay.

· ·

RACHEL'S STORY Rachel's waters had broken the day before with no signs of labour. She went into the hospital for monitoring, and decided to begin the induction process. As her contractions began, she dilated well, and at her first examination she was 3–4 cm. As time went by, Rachel became a bit distressed, and began shaking uncontrollably—a typical sign of high adrenaline levels. We spoke about her options, and she chose to use gas and air. Her body relaxed immediately, and she settled into a great rhythm, lying on her side and coping really well. She felt like she had things under control again, and she voiced this to me by saying that she was feeling good. The gas got her out of her thinking brain, gave her a great focus and helped to regulate her breathing. Her oxytocin levels began to rise, and before long her contractions were coming regularly, so she was moved to the labour ward.

Traffic Light System

So, to summarise this chapter, I want to share with you the tool I use when teaching about oxytocin and adrenaline in my antenatal courses. I like to use the visual of a traffic light system to help couples see what the effects can be.

It's easy to understand that Red = Stop.

A story I like to share is about a woman from my pregnancy yoga class who was expecting her third child. She was in labour and contracting beautifully, and her parents-in-law arrived to babysit her other children so that her husband could drive her to the hospital. As she went to get her bag, she saw a massive spider on the wall and froze. She was petrified of spiders, and in that moment her whole labour shut down. In the end, it stopped for four hours. She had to send her in-laws home and go back to bed and relax before the contractions returned and she was ready to leave for the hospital again.

It's also really easy to understand that Green = Go.

Once labour begins, if the environment is right and the woman is in her zone, then you will see her progressing. It is easy to observe that contractions are becoming longer and closer together. Her breathing ramps up, she tells you she can feel the difference. She looks different and is aware that it is getting tougher.

However, Amber = Contractions with No Progress.

By far the worst possible place to be is between the two, because she still has enough oxytocin to be producing contractions, but not enough to be progressing. In all honesty, I would rather be with a woman who was producing high enough levels of adrenaline to knock out her contractions altogether, which gives her a break, than if she had some levels of both and was stuck in a scenario of contracting with no dilation.

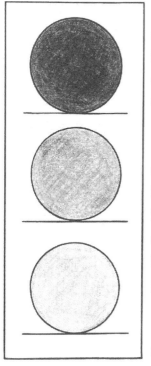

Red = Stop. When a woman has high levels of adrenaline, she cannot be in labour. That's because the powerful effects of adrenaline literally cancel out the effects of oxytocin. High enough levels = no labour.

Amber = Slow Labor. When a woman has some levels of adrenaline, but not enough to knock out oxytocin completely, she will still have contractions. This means that she simply cannot progress as quickly as she should do, because her progress is slowed down by the presence of any adrenaline.

Green = Go. Oxytocin levels are high—labour is in full flow and progressing well.

QUICK RECAP

Here are the main things to remember when discussing hormones.

- **The role of hormones.** Make sure you both understand the role that hormones play during pregnancy and birth, and how each one can impact the process in its own individual way.

- **Be honest!** Talk about how important it is for you to help her protect her oxytocin levels. Consider her personality, and if you have any areas of concern, discuss where you think she may struggle.

- **Plan her labour nest.** Look at the environment where she will spend early labour and gather supplies that can help her relax. These items can include pillows, blankets, headphones, bendy straws, flannels, eye masks and music.

- **Remember the amber light.** Ensure that you both understand any potential issues that could produce adrenaline. Talk about how the amber light in a traffic light is the worst place to be. This can help her to remember how small distractions can often make a big difference to the overall length of labour.

- **Remove distractions.** Arrange suitable childcare or pet care if having others around her in early labour will be distracting.

CHAPTER 5

Dilation

If left alone in labour, the body of a woman produces most easily the baby that is not interfered with by its mother's mind or the assistant's hand. If left alone, just courage and patience are required.

– Grantly Dick-Read

As labour begins, a woman's cervix starts to soften and open, changing from being fully closed to having the ability to stretch to approximately 10 cm in diameter, enabling the baby's head to pass through; this is called dilation. In this chapter, I have broken the process down into three stages. Stage one is the **latent** phase, (meaning early labour); stage two is **dilation**, (when the cervix is opening and labour is established); and stage three is **transition**, (where the cervix has fully opened). I want to make sure that you, as the birth partner, understand the intricacy of these different stages and to know that there is not a one-size-fits-all way that they should happen. All women will experience labour differently, feel the sensations differently, and dilate differently, going through each of the stages at their own pace. It is your job to know that pretty much everything is normal when the body is in charge, and that it is only when interventions are introduced that problems can often arise!

Stage One: The Latent Phase (0–4cm)

Once the baby signals that it is ready to be born, changes to the cervix begin. Progesterone, which has been doing a great job of keeping the cervix tightly closed up to this point, starts to recede, and two essential hormones, prostaglandin and oxytocin, are released. The cervix (the neck of the womb) begins to move forward from its position tucked up towards the back, and it starts to soften and thin out so that it can open (see Figure 5.1). This is an important part of the first stage of labour, which takes some women a few hours and others a few days to complete. As the birth partner, you will need to remember this process can be slow. Remind the woman you are supporting that what is happening deep inside her cannot be rushed, especially if she expresses doubt that labour will ever begin. Any chats you have with her in these last days before birth should be dreamy conversations of the future and of holding and snuggling the baby; any discussions of induction or giving birth in general should be avoided when possible. Make sure you have already covered everything you need to know about your role well in advance, including what items should go in the birth bag, how to call the midwife to the home birth, or how to get to the hospital or MLU. It is also best to avoid speaking to her about your upcoming plans, such as social events, important meetings or appointments, and refrain from drinking alcohol. Mentioning these activities could trigger anxiety or fear that you might not be present and alert for her birth. Above all else, never ever give her a day or time that she should not have the baby. There is nothing worse than being told, even jokingly, to avoid giving birth on a particular date because your birth partner might not be around. You should be available to her unconditionally, even if in the background your life carries on as normal. As a doula, my clients have no idea about what I am doing behind the scenes, as it has no bearing on them. Although I obviously encourage them to give me as much notice as possible, they know I will drop everything the minute they need me. In 20 years I can count on one hand the number of times I have been called out with little to no warning.

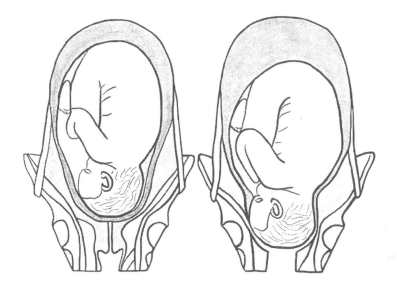

Figure 5.1 The cervix softens, thins and moves out of the way as it is pulled upwards.

Signs of Labour

As the woman you are supporting starts to experience signs of labour, try to keep your excitement to a minimum. There is no doubt that it feels good to know that something is happening, especially if you have been on call for weeks and have been waiting patiently. If labour started at night and is slow to get going by the morning, it may be best to go off to work or go about your regular activities. If she calls you in the daytime to say that she is in labour, do not rush to her; try to stay out of her way and keep occupied. Sitting around all day waiting for labour to ramp up can make her feel like she is under pressure to perform, even if she doesn't realise it. Your excitement or nervousness will rub off on her and she may produce adrenaline. There is nothing you need to do to help her if she is coping well, other than check that she is in a calm and relaxing environment, so if you are around during this stage, it is a good idea to get her settled and comfortable, and then leave her to it. Otherwise, the birth can easily turn into a party, where you end up entertaining each other! When she needs you to be around, she will let you know.

. . . .

JENNIFER'S STORY Jennifer called me at 8 AM to say that she had been labouring for about 5 hours. I asked her how she was feeling, and she said she was excited. She told me that her husband was staying home from work and that they had made plans for their friend to pop over. I knew in that moment that Jennifer would not have the baby that day, and it would be later that night before labour finally took hold. It wasn't until 9 PM, when it was dark outside and Jennifer was alone for the first time all day, that her labour began to ramp up. She started to feel intense contractions by about 10.30 PM and she knew that things had shifted. At our debriefing session a week later, we spoke of how her labour had taken all day to get going, and she admitted that whilst she thought her friend would provide a welcome distraction, in reality, she could see that she felt observed by everyone around her. As the day progressed and her labour didn't, she began to overanalyse what was happening. As soon as she told her husband she was off to bed for an early night, her thoughts and expectations diminished, and her oxytocin levels rose, leading to stronger contractions.

. . . .

The Mucus Plug

One of the first signs of labour for some women is the loss of the mucus plug, often referred to as a 'show'. It can be streaked or tinged with blood; this is perfectly normal and a clear sign that the cervix is working well to prepare for birth. The loss of the mucus plug can happen as early as a week or more before labour begins. (Sex can also cause a bloody discharge, so do check in to see if she might be experiencing this instead). The important thing to do during this time is to go with the flow, and try not to ask too many questions, as this will encourage overthinking. If you are her spouse or family member, and you live with her, you will have the additional benefit of watching her behaviour yourself. She may begin to nest and prepare for the baby, showing an abundance of energy, or alternatively, she may start to instinctively wrap herself in a protective bubble and withdraw from the world. Avoid telling her to 'just relax'. Trust me: this is not helpful. You are better off giving her suggestions of tasks she could do to help her switch off and distract her. Try to think of things you know she will enjoy. One of my clients found that planning a dinner party for her closest friends was a great way to distract herself, sharing that she threw herself into lovingly preparing the meal—whilst another tripped into labour after attending a surprise baby shower that had been scheduled for her around the time of her due date. Some women may prefer a special day out to a gallery or museum, and others might want to curl up with a new book.

Contractions

As the cervix prepares to open, the woman will begin to feel contractions (often referred to as 'surges', 'rushes', 'tightenings' or 'waves'). The cervix is working hard, and the woman can easily become exhausted if she does too much too soon. If she feels like her progress is slow, and she wishes she could speed up labour, remind her again of all the magical changes that are happening inside, and of how incredibly important it is to rest and go with the natural flow of labour. There is no rush, no time limit, no pressure! Whilst this is easy to say, it can be difficult for a woman who likes control, and she may struggle to switch off her thoughts and get into the zone. There is also a tendency for her to become excited or nervous, which can introduce adrenaline. Do your best to say only encouraging things like: 'your body is amazing' or 'trust your body', whilst ensuring she is eating nourishing food, keeping hydrated and getting as much sleep/ rest as possible. Expect to see very inconsistent contractions with no real pattern during the latent phase. You should be able to easily tell that the contractions are irregular—there is no need to time them or write them down, as this makes even the most experienced birth partner want to analyse them. Any discussions about her progress at this stage can set labour back dramatically, so try and stay out of the way as much as possible and say very little.

Turning Contractions

The position of the baby at this time can make a difference to the length of labour. Some women appear to have what I call 'turning contractions'. The baby may need to turn from a posterior position, where the baby's head and back is near its mother's spine, to an anterior one where the baby's spine is closer to the front. The back of the baby's head will then press on the cervix more evenly, which helps it open. Turning contractions tend to be longer than regular contractions and may last up to 1.5 - 2 minutes, sometimes coming in clusters.

Websites like **spinningbabies.com** can show women and their partners positions to adopt that can encourage the baby to move. I recommend the side-lying release and forward-leaning inversion. You can visit the website and practice these positions in advance of the birth, to familiarise yourselves with the concepts, and then if necessary refer back to this on the day if you need to. A typical scenario in the latent phase: a woman thinks that she is in established labour because her contractions are long, only to arrive at the hospital to be told her cervix has only dilated to 1 cm. This can be very disappointing, and she is likely to be sent home. If you think she is experiencing turning contractions in early labour, the best way to manage them is by adopting a forward-leaning position, keeping the baby off the mother's spine, and resting and 'flopping' between every contraction—softening the jaw and shoulders, letting go of all tension, closing the eyes and trusting in the body. You'll find that if the woman can breathe through this phase, her baby will move and her contractions will eventually change: they should in fact slow down, shorten and regularise, giving her a good break between. A reminder that her body is clever and knows how to turn her baby may be all she needs to hear during this time .

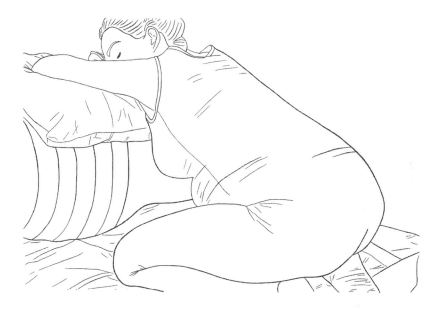

Figure 5.2 Leaning over a peanut ball, a pile of cushions or the edge of a sofa or chair can be really comfortable and can help babies turn if the woman is leaning forward and relaxed between contractions.

'Waters' Breaking

Around 10% of women will experience their waters releasing as the first sign of labour. This happens when the membranes around the baby that contain the amniotic fluid break, and the fluid either trickles out in a steady flow, or gushes out following a 'pop'. You'll know it's the waters breaking when liquid continues to leak out for the duration of labour and birth. Encourage her to put on a sanitary pad, as each time the baby moves, the fluid usually continues leaking out. For most women, around 70%, contractions will begin shortly after their waters break, usually within 24 hours.

She should take note of the following: Colour, Odour, Amount, and Time (in an easy-to-remember acronym, COAT).

- **Colour.** Her waters should be clear. Yellow or greenish-brown could indicate the baby has had a bowel movement (meconium). A thick dark brown colour can indicate the baby is in distress.
- **Odour.** A mild or odourless smell is normal, but a strong odour might indicate infection.
- **Amount.** Note whether it is a trickle or a gush.
- **Time.** There is an increased risk of infection as time passes once her waters break, so the midwife will ask for this information to record it in her notes.

Whilst it is recommended that a woman contacts the midwife or hospital to let them know what is happening, she should remember that an offer to come to the hospital is just that—an offer. She can have a discussion with the midwife on duty about what her options include, perhaps choosing to stay home for a while longer. For example, if her waters broke in the middle of the night, and she wasn't worried, she might decide to go back to bed for a while, giving her oxytocin levels a chance to rise automatically. If, however, by morning, she still hasn't felt any contractions, then a trip to the hospital might be a reasonable thing to do if she is concerned. If she does elect to go, she may be advised to have an examination or swab test to confirm that her waters have broken, and they will also want to monitor the baby. Ideally vaginal examinations (VE) should be kept to a minimum, or declined completely at this stage as they increase the risk of infection for the woman. Sexual intercourse is also an infection risk and is not advised after her waters have broken. If labour doesn't begin within 24 to 48 hours, she will be invited to attend the hospital for an induction of labour (see Chapter 15). Again this should be seen as just a recommendation, and not all women will choose to accept it. If she does decline induction, she can discuss this with the hospital and work out how they will continue to monitor her moving forward. Monitoring can include her taking her own temperature regularly, avoiding all vaginal examinations, keeping a record of her baby's movements and observing her amniotic fluid.

Premature Rupture of Membranes (PROM)

If a woman's waters break prematurely (before 37 weeks), and there are no signs of labour, she may be advised to have an induction. If there is not an immediate health risk to her or the baby, and she would prefer not to be induced, she can have a conversation with the doctor about continuing the pregnancy until the baby is ready to be born. In this instance, she may be offered routine use of antibiotics to keep the risk of infection low. This is called 'prophylactic' use, and is intended to prevent infection from developing; however, it is not a guarantee. As there are also side effects to both mother and baby from routine use of antibiotics in labour and birth, I recommend you both do some research, before she decides to accept or decline. If she does decide to go ahead with antibiotics, then she should consider taking a good quality probiotic in the early postnatal period (see Chapter 16), for both her and the baby. The woman may also be offered steroids at this time, which are given to mature her baby's lungs in case labour begins and the baby is born sooner than expected.

· ·

KAYLIE'S STORY Kaylie called me at 35 weeks to let me know her waters had broken. She went to the hospital to be checked and was feeling really scared. Her doctor had told her that they were not sure if the baby would trigger labour, but if there were still no signs after 24 hours they would begin an induction. Kaylie felt she would prefer to wait until the labour started on its own, so I recommended that she read the NICE guidelines on her phone in the hospital. She then had a conversation with the doctor about remaining pregnant, and they made the decision together that Kaylie would go home and wait. Kaylie's labour started three weeks later, at 38 weeks and two days. After daily monitoring of her temperature, and no vaginal examinations in order to avoid the risk of infection, she had a completely normal birth and was delighted that she had avoided induction.

. . . .

Stage Two: Dilation (up to 9 cm)

For most women, this is the 'established phase' where contractions will begin in earnest. These might be felt anywhere from her breasts to her knees. I would usually expect to hear that the sensations are coming from her lower abdomen or lower back, but it can often vary. I have had a few clients who have not realised that they were in labour because the sensations weren't the period-type pains that had been described to them in their antenatal classes. One client had been feeling constipated all day and was surprised to discover that she was in established labour after alerting her midwife that she thought something was wrong. She had emptied her bowels several times, but the sensations to her were the same as feeling constipated, which was why she never suspected labour. Some women have told me that they felt their contractions in the tops of their legs, so be prepared for any variations.

Dilation Chart

I have been using this chart (see Figure 5.3) for many years when teaching couples about dilation. The circles represent the process of dilation, from 0 to 10 cm. As you look at the circles, you might imagine that all women have to pass through each and every number to get to 10. I have removed these numbers, because I do not believe they are relevant at all. The fact is that one woman might go from 1 to 10 very quickly, whilst another might remain at 4 for many hours, before slowly progressing to 10. Giving birth is not a race. It's not a competition to see who can get there the fastest. There is no straightforward direct route, and many may experience a plateau for longer periods than others. Instead, I like to encourage women to avoid thinking of numbers at all.

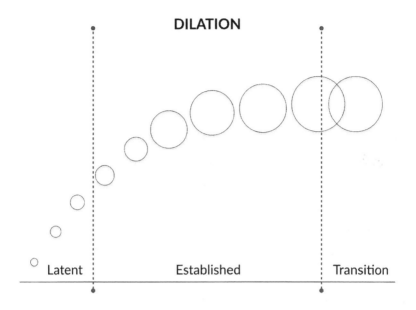

Figure 5.3 Dilation Chart. The circles represent the opening of the cervix from 1 to 10 cm. As the sensations intensify and the contractions get closer together, there are smaller rest periods in between. (Based on original by Pam England from her book *Birthing from Within*.)

As you look at the chart, you might notice that somewhere in the middle, the circles get bigger and are closer together. In reality, contractions may not get more intense after this stage, but may begin to last longer with the gaps between getting smaller. The need to rest between contractions becomes very important. It's common for many women when they reach this halfway point in labour to have a confidence dip, believing they cannot cope anymore. Lots of women will have a good cry and need a hug. Keep telling her she is amazing, and if she doesn't use her safety word, keep going.

Resting Between Contractions

Contractions are intermittent: they come and go, which gives the woman an opportunity to recover and take a break. As each one eases off, she should rest and 'flop' (release all her muscles), giving her the chance to conserve her energy for as long as labour takes. In this phase, expect the contractions to last for anywhere between 20 and 40 seconds, ramping up to nearer 60 seconds in length as labour progresses. At this time, ensure that the environment is optimal. Prepare the room with oxytocin in mind: dark, warm, quiet, safe. Each time she completes the contraction, observe her behavior. Whilst it is important not to say much at this stage or be too 'coachy', she may need a gentle reminder to relax and soften. It is difficult to know how long the gap will be between surges, as some women (like myself) have contractions with short gaps from the outset, and others will form the more typical pattern that begins with big gaps that get smaller and smaller over time. Contractions can be very irregular in early labour, but as they do begin to regularise, you will see them change in the following ways.

- **Strength.** The way she is coping with them may begin to change when the surges intensify.
- **Length.** They will start to lengthen the more oxytocin she is producing. You will both be able to easily tell the difference between a 30-second and a 60-second contraction.
- **Distance Between.** They will begin to creep closer together. You may notice they begin to form a pattern. You can literally set your watch by them. This is a good sign that labour is becoming established. Don't jump up after this has happened a few times, as you will still have some way to go yet, but you can feel confident that when a pattern begins to form she is leaving the latent phase and creeping into the established phase.

Positions

I have written a whole chapter on positions (see Chapter 8) to give you ideas about what positions are useful to adopt at each stage of labour, wherever you might be. It is vital that the woman remains comfortable and rested between contractions from beginning to end where possible, which assists the production of oxytocin. Her instincts can play a huge role when it comes to alignment of the baby in her pelvis and it is interesting how she will often adopt a position without even realising that it's helping to create more room. I was at a home birth many years ago where the mother would lift and stretch out her right leg on to the arm of the sofa with every contraction. She clearly needed to make some extra space on that side of her pelvis for the baby. When we spoke about it afterwards, she was completely unaware that she had been doing it.

When to Make the Call

The universal recommendation for when to call a midwife to your home birth, or leave for the hospital, is when the contractions are:

* Coming regularly and forming a pattern,
* Consistently lasting about a minute, and
* Coming about three times in every 10 minutes.

Whilst there will come a point where you might want to know the timings of her contractions, to indeed confirm that she is having at least three in every 10 minutes, and that they are lasting about a minute, it is my recommendation that you do not time them throughout the entire labour. The information is completely irrelevant, and can rob the woman of her chance to relax. You, as the birth partner, may end up too focused on the timings and not be present enough for her, or she might be aware of what you're doing and be too tempted to analyse them herself. When you are beginning to think that the contractions are coming consistently and are definitely lasting longer than they were before, then try counting under your breath to get a rough idea how long each contraction is. If you have counted up to at least 60 seconds, then that is a good gauge. My top tip here is to watch her. Sit somewhere in the room where she cannot see you, and observe her behaviour. If the contraction ends and she springs back to normal, she is not ready. She may be vocalising that she is finding them tough, but what you are looking for in her behaviour is a long recovery period after the contraction has ended: a noticeable sign that she is going inward. She should not really be aware that you are around her. You should quietly offer her a sip of water every two to three contractions, and a bite to eat every hour or so, but other than that, just sit quietly and close by. When she does ask you to make the call, and you think she is ready, time the contractions unobtrusively for 10 minutes and record the information to share with the midwife over the telephone. If she is not quite at the point where you think you should call, then just keep going with the flow. If she asks you if you think it's nearly time, tell her that you will call shortly, but you think she is doing so well at the moment that you don't want to set her back. As long as she is managing the contractions and the baby is moving regularly, your intention is to help the oxytocin loop for a bit longer, getting her past the point of no return.

IMPORTANT TO KNOW   *If this is a second or subsequent baby, then dilation can happen quickly, so you should consider calling a midwife earlier in the process outlined above, especially if the contractions are regular and consistent in length.*

Feel her Legs

One of the ways I try to identify if a woman is progressing in labour is to feel her legs. As all the blood is heading to the uterus, and away from the limbs, the temperature of her legs usually changes.

I tend to gauge it this way:

* If her legs are warm but her feet and ankles are cold, then I assume her cervix is approximately three cm dilated.
* If her legs are cold up to perhaps the mid-calf area, she is probably around five cm.
* If her legs up to the knee are cold, she may be fully dilated.

Making the Call

Most hospitals have a telephone triage system: an over-the-phone assessment that will try and ascertain if she is indeed ready to receive support from a midwife. Even an MLU, or home birth team, will want to ask a few questions about what is happening with the woman, so have answers to the following questions ready before you pick up the phone.

* How frequent are the contractions?
* How long are they lasting?
* Have her waters broken and if so what time? What did they look like?
* How is she coping?

Take the phone as far away from the woman as you can, so that she doesn't hear the conversation. Assuming the midwife is fine talking to you as her birth partner, you can describe your circumstances and then if they agree that she is ready, you can pack up the car to drive her in, or wait for the 'on-call' midwife to arrive at the home. They may prefer to speak to the woman personally, to gauge how advanced they think the labour might be. The midwife will keep her talking and will listen to see if she has any contractions while they are on the phone with her, and how she copes when she does. If a woman is low-risk, the midwife on the phone will always encourage her to stay at home for as long as possible. If she is hypnobirthing, be sure to mention this to the midwife, as a woman who is calm and relaxed can often be mistaken for a woman in early labour. If she is considered high-risk, she might be asked to come into the hospital much earlier in labour. This is usually discussed with the woman in advance, so it may already be something you are aware of.

Seeking Advice

Feel free to call the midwife to ask for some advice, especially if there is something you are concerned about. If at that time they recommend that you bring the woman in to hospital, remember this might just be standard advice and not specific to the woman you are supporting. You can have a reasonable discussion with the midwife about the pros and cons of this before the woman decides what to do. An example might be that the woman you are supporting has lost her mucus plug, and it is quite bloody. It's a heavy red mucus rather than bright red blood running down her legs, and you are unsure if that is normal. They could propose that you bring her in, mentioning that they are not overly busy and might as well make sure that any blood loss isn't a concern. Midwives are just doing their job in suggesting this, but a trip into hospital at this stage could change the outcome of the birth, so be clear from the outset whether you are looking for supportive advice and reassurance or you are genuinely worried.

Always Believe the Woman

I want you to know that a woman's instinct trumps everything. In my experience, if a woman is progressing quickly, and she tells you that something is happening, she is usually right. This does not include a woman who is wondering if she should call the midwife; this is a woman who is telling you she definitely should.

From Home to Hospital

Transporting a woman in labour is a big responsibility! Having done it many times (in a tiny Fiat 500!), I recommend the following.

- Plan your route well in advance. You won't want to use a navigation system unless it's on silent.
- Be aware of the time of day you leave, avoiding rush hour where possible.
- Make sure she is comfortable in whatever position she can find.
- Don't drive too fast even though she will want you to make the journey as quickly as possible.
- Stay calm and drive safely, especially if she is not secured in a seatbelt. And remember that any bump in the road you can feel may be even more uncomfortable to her!
- If possible, try to avoid arriving just before or around the time of a shift change when the staff are busy doing handovers. These are usually anytime between 7 AM–8.30 AM and 7 PM–8.30 PM.

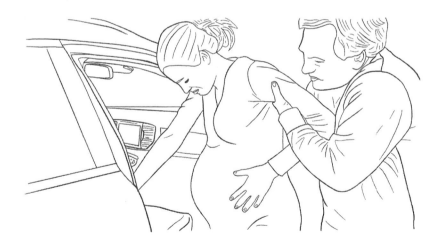

Home Birth Withdrawal

It is not uncommon for a birth partner to call the hospital when the woman is in established labour, asking for the midwife to attend them at home, and be told that there is no one available. You would then be informed that you have to bring the woman into the hospital or MLU to give birth instead of staying home as arranged. In this instance you will need to be very strong, and ask to speak to the on-call duty manager. A planned home birth has been booked in, and the service should not be withdrawn in the event that the unit is short-staffed. Sadly, this is a common occurrence in the UK, and it is important to be firm in this instance. The midwife in charge should be able to find a replacement midwife to send out to you if you refuse to leave home and travel in.

· ·

JOANNAH'S STORY   Joannah was in labour with her fourth baby and was booked for a homebirth. She had been clear from the outset that her plan was to give birth at home, so she was shocked on the day to be told she would need to go into the unit as there was no one available to attend. The midwife on the end of the phone was adamant that she was unable to send anyone out. After a chat with Joannah to see how she felt, her doula was able to explain calmly to the midwife that Joannah would be staying at home and required support. Less than 10 minutes later, two midwives arrived at the door.

· ·

Face-to-Face Support

As soon as you arrive at the chosen place of birth, or a midwife arrives at home, the midwife will want to see the woman's pregnancy notes, and any other paperwork she has, including the birth plan (see Chapter 13). The midwife will typically ask to perform a set of observations on the woman, which usually involves checking her blood pressure and pulse and possibly requesting a urine sample. They will also ask to listen to the baby's heartbeat and have a feel of the woman's belly to check the position of the baby. At this point she will also be offered a vaginal examination.

Monitoring the Baby During Labour

Wherever a woman chooses to give birth within the UK, once she is in established labour and her intrapartum care begins ('intrapartum' meaning within or during labour), the standard guidance is for her midwife to listen in to the baby's heart rate every 15 minutes during the first stage (dilation), and every five minutes during the second stage (pushing). This is called 'intermittent auscultation'. By listening to the baby's heart rate regularly, the midwife will have an idea of the baby's baseline heartrate, which can indicate whether the baby is coping well with each contraction. Midwives are looking for a good variability between 110 bpm and 160 bpm. Below 110 bpm is called bradycardia (abnormally slow heart rate) and above 160 bpm is called tachycardia (very rapid heart rate). A baby who is continually going above or below the baseline is thought to be showing signs of distress.

There are three options for monitoring available for women giving birth at home or in an MLU:

1. Pinard. The midwife can use a trumpet-like stethoscope called a 'pinard'. It is a hollow horn, typically made of wood, and used to amplify sound. First, the midwife will feel for the position of the baby using their hands (palpation). They will then place the pinard on the woman's belly, and put their ear at the opening in order to listen to the baby's heart rate. This method does not allow the mother to hear; however, it is not invasive for the baby, so many women prefer it. It takes great skill and practice to use a pinard, which is often used in addition to a doppler.

2. Fetoscope. A fetoscope is very much like a regular stethoscope, except that it has a bell-shaped end which magnifies the sound waves of the fetal heart and can be heard by the person using the device. Many independent midwives use this option when listening to the baby, and might encourage family members and any older children to have a listen as well.

3. Doppler or **Sonicaid.** Alternatively, midwives carry a 'doppler' (an ultrasound device that acts like a speaker) with them at all times. Most are waterproof so can be used if a woman gives birth in a birth pool. This is the same device used to listen to babies during an antenatal appointment, so the woman you are supporting should be very familiar with this form of monitoring. Each time the midwife listens to the baby, it is a requirement that the midwife seek permission from the woman to make sure that she consents before the midwife is able to touch her with the device. For many women, this can be incredibly disruptive and will continually bring them out of the labour zone they are in. I always suggest to clients who are happy for the midwife to listen to the baby regularly that they might like to give blanket permission. That way the midwife can come and kneel beside the woman and can listen to the baby's heart rate without having to ask. As long as the midwife is quiet and unobtrusive and keeps the sound of the doppler turned down, the woman tends not to be too disturbed. In some cases, a woman can find that every 15 minutes is just too invasive, and she can ask for larger gaps in between. Whilst every 15 minutes is a recognised guideline across the country, it is not evidence-based. As midwife Rachel Reed points out on her website, **midwifethinking.com**: 'There is NO research to date examining whether the practice of fetal heart rate auscultation is beneficial, or the optimal frequency of auscultation. There may be theoretical and experiential evidence to support the practice, but the timing seems to have been plucked out of the air and set in stone.' It is hard to know how the woman you are supporting will feel about regular monitoring until the day itself, but definitely have a discussion about it during the antenatal period to gain a sense of what her immediate thoughts are. Some women have really strong opinions from the outset, whereas others take a more flexible approach.

IMPORTANT TO KNOW   *If the woman is in water, midwives might occasionally forget to switch the doppler off when they are placing the device under the water. It makes a really loud screeching sound when that happens, so feel free to remind the midwife to switch the device on only when it is in place.*

4. Electronic Fetal Monitoring. If a woman is in the main labour ward, or a large obstetric unit, possibly because she is high risk, then she may be offered electronic fetal monitoring (EFM). This particular monitor has wires attached to circular disks that are strapped to the woman's belly using stretchy belts. They provide a continuous trace of the baby's heart rate, and they also measure the woman's contractions. This option usually involves the woman having to remain in one place, which can make it hard for her to mobilise as the straps around her tummy can slip and move. This makes the experience of wearing the belts uncomfortable and problematic. Again, there is no evidence to suggest that EFM is beneficial, except that it is shown to significantly increase the likelihood of c-sections and assisted birth. It is therefore useful for a woman to know that she can decline EFM if she chooses. If she does consent, think about covering the machine with a jacket and turning the sound down. Otherwise you will both sit and watch the monitor, which can have a hugely negative effect on hormone production. You could also ask if the hospital has a wireless version, called 'telemetry', which will help her get into a more comfortable upright position free from restrictions. She can go to the toilet with it on or get into the pool. If the woman has an epidural, however, the monitor will be required to be on at all times so the midwife can ensure the baby is coping well with the drug. This has little impact on the woman as she cannot move around by then anyway (see Chapter 12 for more information on birth management).

IMPORTANT TO KNOW   *Sometimes, as the baby moves, the trace can be lost and parents can start to panic. The midwife in this instance will come and reposition the disk. Also, there may be some changes to the heart rate pattern (decelerations) towards the end of the pushing stage, as the baby is being* *compressed in the birth canal. As long as the heart rate recovers quickly, this is normal even though it can be worrying to listen to.*

5. Fetal Scalp Electrode. In the instance that a good trace cannot easily be found when the woman is wearing an EFM, and there are concerns about how the baby is coping, the woman may be asked if she agrees to have a fetal scalp electrode (FSE) clipped onto the top of her baby's head. This is a way to monitor the heart rate continuously and can only be placed after the waters have broken. There will be a thin wire left between the woman's legs that attaches to the monitor. Some women prefer this method, because it gives them a little more freedom than the EFM belts. A woman must always make a decision based on informed choice for the specific situation she is facing at that time.

IMPORTANT TO KNOW   *This method of monitoring will scratch the baby's scalp, so there is a small risk of infection to the baby*

Checking for Progress

A vaginal examination (VE) is an intimate procedure where the midwife or doctor inserts two fingers into the pregnant woman's vagina and feels for dilation and condition of the cervix. I always offer a word of caution here, because VEs are not always accurate and do carry risks. (Please read the detailed discussion in Chapter 14). Once a woman has had a VE, she is (according to hospital guidelines) expected to have another every four hours throughout labour, but hospitals don't try very hard to inform you that a VE is optional. In my opinion this is because midwives and doctors are trained to use this common assessment tool over and above other physiological signs and rely on it too heavily. They often don't take the time to observe the woman closely and cannot tell how progressed she is during her labour without performing a VE. If, however, the woman herself wants to know if she is making progress and feels the information will be valuable to her, then consenting to the VE is fine, as long as she isn't accepting just because she doesn't realise she can decline. It is also not unusual for a woman who has expressed a preference to avoid routine VEs in the antenatal period to change her own mind in the moment. In this instance, if she says she has changed her mind, double check with her that she is sure, especially if you think she is tired and being compliant, as she could be set back both emotionally and physiologically if it looks like she's dilated by a low number of centimeters. Midwife Sara Wickham calls this 'cervical recoil'. If this is the case, you might suggest she wait an hour before she accepts, so that she has the opportunity to adjust to her new surroundings and feel more comfortable.

Failure to Progress vs Failure to be Patient

In my experience, too many assessments can lead to a diagnosis of 'failure to progress' (a term used for slow labour when an intervention is recommended). Current guidelines in the UK suggest that a woman should show progress by dilating at least one cm every two hours. As I mentioned earlier in this chapter, a woman is unlikely to dilate in exact numerical order and may stick at four cm for a while then jump to seven cm. Many women will plateau at some point during labour, and speed up at others. Avoiding VEs will eliminate the likelihood that her midwife will check her twice during a plateau and find there has been no further dilation. If that happens, she may be told that she needs help to speed up her contractions, as they are not efficiently opening her cervix. This can lead to a complete decline in her positivity and a premature switch to Plan B.

Being labelled in this way can lead to doubt in future pregnancies too, with the word 'failure' hanging over the woman. So rather than the using the phrase 'failure to progress', I prefer to call this 'failure to be patient' on the part of the care providers. If the woman herself is not requesting to be checked, then my advice is to leave well enough alone. If she is okay, and the baby is okay, then it is more useful to encourage her to let go of the need to keep checking, and do as little as possible other than to be producing an abundance of hormones and adopt a good position. If the woman you are supporting is really keen to know what her dilation progress is, then of course having a VE is a good decision for her. Once the examination is over, she can then either put that thought behind her and move on, or, if she is ready to make a new plan because she feels what she has been doing is no longer working for her, then it is a good time to do so.

Her Body, Her Choice!

As her birth partner, you may have asked for a safety word to be in place (see Chapter 3), which will help you know if she definitely wants to move forward in a new direction. If she uses the safety word, it is important that you are prepared to switch to Plan B. Even if you are disappointed, try not to show it. Women will often share that they were ready to give up, but they didn't want to disappoint their birth partner, so they carried on and regretted it. A safety word will eliminate this issue, so be sure to encourage the woman you are supporting to choose one.

Stage Three: Transition (9–10 cm)

Transition is a magical time and worth keeping an eye out for. As her body is shifting from the unconscious to the conscious, she begins to wake up! The parasympathetic nervous system is being taken over by the sympathetic nervous system, and the woman is experiencing a hit of adrenaline. As she enters fight or flight mode, she may begin to have moments of doubt as her brain starts to re-engage. She might look you in the eye and tell you that she definitely cannot go on; she might accuse you of not helping her; and she may even say her safety word. If this happens to you, and you suspect she is in transition, then you may have to check in with her and perhaps even discuss the option of a VE to make sure she doesn't switch to Plan B in error. A textbook transitional phase will see her go from contracting beautifully, to asking for an epidural, then straight into involuntary pushing, often before that VE is performed. This is not the case for all women, however, and the length of this stage can vary. (I will cover more about transition in Chapter 6).

QUICK RECAP

Here are the main things to remember when discussing dilation.

- **Don't chase the labour!** Try to encourage her to rest during labour as much as possible. An active birth means don't lie on the bed on your back; it doesn't mean exhaust yourself trying to chase the labour.

- **Eat and drink as normal.** She should eat well during labour and drink constantly. Water is essential and should be offered after every two or three contractions. (See Chapter 9 for ideas on snacks and drinks).

- **She should empty her bladder regularly.** The bladder can fill during labour and restrict the room that the baby has to move down, so regular visits to the toilet are important. I recommend every hour or two.

- **Rest and flop between contractions.** Adopting a comfortable position is essential to maintain labour for the long haul, and to keeping oxytocin levels high.

- **Let your monkey do it!** Ina May Gaskin, an American lay midwife, talks about letting the 'monkey mind' get into its primitive state, which involves not overthinking everything. This is good advice for dilation.

CHAPTER 6

Pushing

Giving birth should be your greatest achievement, not your greatest fear.
–Jane Weideman

Midwives and doctors are taught in medical school how the baby rotates through its mother's pelvis during the process of birth, and current textbooks state that it is better for the woman, especially a first-time mother, to push in an upright position. All childbirth experts understand that by remaining upright and using the additional effects of gravity, with the benefits of the hormone relaxin, a woman's sacrum (the triangular bone at the base of the spine) and coccyx (tailbone) have the ability to lift and move out of the way, creating up to 30% more space in the pelvis for the baby to pass through. Despite this, medical professionals are still only taught how to examine a woman lying on her back, which can be problematic for many reasons. Once a woman gets onto a bed to be examined in labour, research shows she is highly likely to remain there, despite the fact that it can make labour more painful. This is due to the excess abdominal weight of the uterus on the spine and coccyx, which can put pressure on important blood vessels, possibly compromising blood flow to the baby. The combination of both restrictions on movement and the pelvis being unable to open to its maximum capacity, can lead to the likelihood of more interventions. Whilst it might be easier for the care provider, as they can see the vagina more clearly, it is definitely not good for the mother or the baby. In fact, it is well documented that a woman who pushes out her baby when lying down or in a semi-recumbent position, is more likely to require support, with the list of interventions increasing as the woman struggles to give birth. By discussing the issue antenatally and encouraging the mother to stay off her back in both the first and second stages of labour, the birth partner can help to facilitate both comfort for the woman and a more direct route through the birth canal for the baby.

IMPORTANT TO KNOW   If she is happy to lie on the bed for a vaginal examination, encourage her to get up quickly, before the midwife or doctor discusses the results with her. This can be beneficial both mentally and physically, and she will be at their eye level when talking rather than remaining in a very vulnerable position laying supine on the bed. This can help her to feel more in control of any decisions that may be made at that point.

What's wrong with this picture?

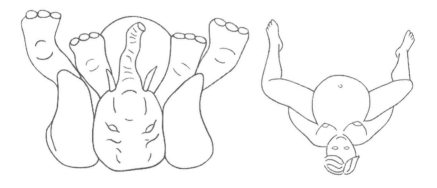

Stephanie Larson from Dancing for Birth produced this image in 2010, showing an elephant lying on its back. She said 'Imagine trying to restrict an elephant to give birth on her back. It would probably require drugs and might lead to surgery'.

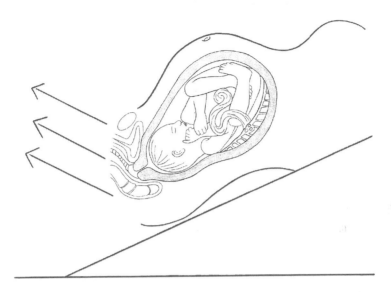

Most women who give birth on their backs will be in this position—semi-recumbent—rather than lying completely flat. The woman has to push her baby down, and then up, before the baby can emerge.

I have to admit that I was a woman who gave birth lying on my back the first time around. There was no mention of me being in an upright position, and I hadn't realised when I had an epidural that I would be so restricted being attached to a monitor. I found the pushing stage horrendous because I didn't know what I was doing as I couldn't feel a thing. After a couple of hours of coached pushing, I had burst blood vessels in my eyes, haemorrhoids in my bum, and I was exhausted with nothing left in me. In the end I had an episiotomy to help get my son out, as he was becoming distressed, and the infant resuscitation team ran into the room to help him. He was fine, but was taken away from me to be checked over and was then passed to my husband and my mother before I was able to hold him almost 45 minutes later, due to me requiring stitches. This exact scenario had been my worst fear, but at the time I was so relieved that it was over, I didn't really consider the lasting implications on both my body and my relationship with my baby. It was only when I was pregnant again two years later that I began to fully understand how much intervention I had received due to the position I had pushed in, and what impact that had on those early postnatal months as my body slowly recovered. It was at this time that my journey to becoming a doula began, as I started to learn how clever women's bodies are, and how they are designed to give birth away from beds and medical equipment.

Back to Transition

So let's just go back for a minute and pretend that the woman is only just entering transition. She is still having regular contractions, but something is changing.

What happens next could be one of the following.

- She feels an urge to push only at the peak of a contraction.
- She feels an urge to push every now and again, but not all the time.
- She describes an urge to push but is not pushing.

All of these signal that she still has some dilating to do. Leave her and give her encouragement if she needs it. Sometimes a snack at this time works really well, and a trip to the toilet encouraging her to stay for a while if you can, which can offer privacy whilst also creating extra room in her pelvis as she sits on the toilet bowl.

If the following are true:

- She falls asleep and her contractions become spaced out, or
- Her contractions stop completely for a while

then this is a sign of the 'rest and be thankful stage'—a natural lull in labour—so let her rest. DO NOT wake her up. Leave her alone and feel confident that her body knows exactly what it is doing.

When she starts to feel an overwhelming urge to push from the beginning of every single contraction, which she couldn't stop if she tried, you can feel confident that she is entering the second stage of labour. She should follow her body and go with what she is feeling. If necessary, encourage her to tune in and let her body take over. If anyone tries to direct her during this time, remind her to 'follow her body's natural urge'.

Signs of Full Dilation

When a woman is fully dilated, there is usually a noticeable purple line that has grown up the natal cleft—the deep groove which runs between the two buttocks (also known as the butt crack). As labour begins, this line starts at the anal margin, and creeps up like a thermometer. When it reaches the top, the woman is 10 cm dilated (see Figure 6.3). This happens when an increase in pressure causes congestion in the veins around the sacrum. It

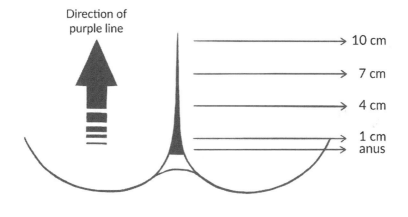

Figure 6.3

is not noticeable in all women but it is worth looking out for if the woman you are supporting is on her hands and knees and her lower back and buttocks are visible. Other signs include feeling the urge to vomit as the pressure in her body builds, or feeling flushed and very warm. Her lower legs may feel cold and she may begin to tremble as a surge of adrenaline arrives to wake her up and give her the energy to push.

Rest and Be Thankful

The late natural birth advocate and author Sheila Kitzinger always offered great wisdom in her various books. One of her many observations about physiological birth is that some women will experience what she calls a 'rest and be thankful' stage. This is a period of time that can occur between the first and second stages of labour, when there is a temporary lull and contractions slow down or stop altogether. The woman may fall asleep and really benefit from the break. At this stage, midwives often fear the labour may have stalled, when in fact it is simply the body's way of giving the uterus a moment to gather itself before going in for the big push. If you notice the contractions start to space out, or tail off for a period of time, your job is to encourage her to rest. She needs to switch off her brain and let go of any tension in her body. Her uterus knows exactly what it is doing, and it will soon kick back into action again.

IMPORTANT TO KNOW   If at any time during an obvious 'rest and be thankful' stage, the midwife or doctor suggests a synthetic oxytocin drip to bring back the contractions, I recommend you ask if she can have an hour to rest first. In my experience, the wait usually does the trick and the contractions come back on their own.

Going for a Poo

One of the ways I talk about the pushing stage in my classes is to get the attendees to think about what the sensations of needing a poo feel like. If you go to the toilet when you first think that you need to go, you can sit there for a while before you are actually ready to poo. If you wait and wait and wait until you are desperate, however, you can go and be done quickly. This is exactly the same advice for a woman pushing out a baby—she should wait, so she will be able to work quickly and efficiently with her body. Another example I share is about how the need to go to the toilet can be stalled by something happening. Perhaps you are heading to a 9:00 AM meeting. You have been stuck in the car or on the train, and you know you need to go, but you won't have time before the meeting begins. Once your mind becomes distracted, the sensation will usually disappear. The need to go may return immediately after the meeting, or it may wait for an appropriate time later that day when it feels safe and in some cases will only return when you walk in your front door at home. Similarly, if the labouring woman is distracted by an external influence that derails her labour, the urge to push can be delayed for many hours, as an adrenaline surge will send all the blood to her limbs to prepare her to run from danger (see Ginny's story). Sometimes I ask one of my course attendees to participate in an experiment where I ask them to squat down in the middle of the floor and push out a poop. I give them five minutes, and tell them we will all watch. I will also check in every minute and shine a bright torch on their anus to see if I can see progress. As you can imagine, no one ever agrees to take part. Do you think they would be able to go? Unlikely I suspect. All of this is to help them understand the conditions a woman is in when she is expected to push out a baby with her vagina on display, surrounded by strangers. Her sphincter muscles can get a little shy if the conditions are not optimal, and she feels under pressure or overly exposed. If she misses this window, she may need to relax and wait for the sensations to return.

Fetus Ejection Reflex

The pushing phase is an extremely important part of the birthing process, and it can be easy or hard, depending on the woman's understanding of how involuntary that process is when it is completely physiological. By trusting that her body will tell her when the time is right, she will be able to work with an internal force that is designed to push the baby out—a mechanism a bit like vomiting. French obstetrician and childbirth specialist Michel Odent speaks of a huge surge of adrenaline that the woman can experience at this exact point in labour, which wakes her up and helps to expel the baby quickly and efficiently. This is called 'the fetus ejection reflex'. Unlike vomiting, however, this reflex is pretty delicate, and the minute an outside influence arises and distracts the woman, this reflex and its benefits can be lost. Some women are more sensitive to their immediate environment than others at this stage. It is therefore important to assume that the woman you are supporting will be too, and you and anyone else present, should be incredibly mindful of remaining quiet and protective of her space. This is not a good time for her to be offered vaginal examinations, be asked questions, or be given suggestions, as it can delay her from feeling that overwhelming urge to push. Hopefully with the optimal environment, her body will do all the work itself and the baby will be born quickly and easily.

Ticking Clock

If the midwife has documented that the woman has entered the second stage, then the clock will start ticking. In most hospitals, an hour—or possibly up to two at the midwife's discretion—is considered the maximum time a woman is 'allowed' to push before they want to see signs of the baby's head. This means that a woman can literally run out of time, giving her body no chance to push voluntarily. Most midwives will wait until they see the woman show signs of an expulsive pushing urge before they document this stage, but if the woman begins pushing before she is truly ready, or she has a vaginal examination that reveals she is fully dilated, then she can run out of time before the second stage gets going.

· ·

GINNY'S STORY Ginny arrived at the hospital after labouring at home for over 24 hours. She agreed to a VE upon arrival, and it was discovered that she was already fully dilated, but her contractions had diminished. The midwives jumped into action despite this, and behaved as though the baby was coming immediately. Ginny was fine and the baby was fine, but her body was taking a break. We were shown into a labour room, and we ran the birth pool thinking about how relaxing it would be for Ginny to get into the warm water for a while. When the midwife came back 45 minutes later she told us that if there were no signs of Ginny pushing within the next 15 minutes, that they were going to have to intervene. At this point she explained that because Ginny had been given an examination, and her cervix was found to be fully dilated, the clock had started ticking without us knowing. The additional time pressure that Ginny felt meant that there was no chance her body was going to produce contractions. She needed time to relax and for the circumstances to be right, and she simply ran out of time. In the end, the doctor decided Ginny's baby was at risk of developing an infection due to her water's having broken the day before, and her baby was born by c-section. Ginny was devastated.

Pushing for Primips

I always loved the article written by Canadian midwife/birth attendant Gloria Lemay, called 'Pushing for Primips'. I have shared this so many times with clients over the years, and it has been incredibly useful in their understanding of the pushing phase and how to manage it for the first time. Go ahead and give it a read at **wisewomanwayofbirth.com** (see the Resources section at the back of the book). Gloria talks of the need for patience when a woman is pushing out her first baby (primip). She describes the process as 'a space in time where her obstetrical future often gets decided'. She explains that much mischief can take place when a woman feels pressure to perform and begins to push before she is ready. This is a very delicate stage, and she cautions that a vaginal examination at this point can cause a delay in the process. This opinion goes against the medical narrative that a woman should not push until she is found to be fully dilated or she may cause herself harm. If the cervix were to swell, the baby would struggle to be born vaginally. I suspect that if a midwife or doctor has ever discovered a woman with a swollen cervix, it is more likely that it was caused by directed pushing, and not the woman gently pushing instinctively. As Gloria goes on to explain, the final part of dilation and the early pushing stage are vitally important, and no woman ever swelled her own cervix by listening to her body. She speaks of the need for midwives to change their notion of what is happening in the pushing phase with a primip from 'descent of the head' to 'shaping of the head.' Each expulsive sensation shapes the head of the baby to conform to the contours of the mother's pelvis. This can take time and lots of patience.

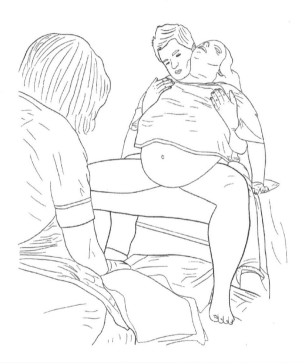

Figure 6.4 This drawing shows the birth partner supporting the woman in a squat by sitting behind her on a chair. This can be a comfortable position for both during the pushing phase.

Pressure to perform

If, for whatever reason, the woman you are supporting consents to having a vaginal examination, or she asks for one and is found to be 9 cm or 10 cm dilated, then everyone in the room, you included, may expect her to begin pushing soon after. It can lead to impatience, with the birth attendants standing around thinking, 'come on then, where are these pushes'? In this instance, and I see it regularly, a woman can end up pushing before she is ready, because she is asked so many times about what she is feeling, she may begin to believe that she should be pushing by now too. You might hear the midwife ask questions like:

- 'Where are you feeling those contractions now?'
- 'Do you feel anything in your bottom?'
- 'Are you feeling a little pushy?' or
- 'You're 10 cm, do you feel like pushing?'

You can understand why a woman in this scenario might begin pushing, even though her body is not actually ready. The problem is, pushing prematurely due to feeling under pressure to perform means she is not working with her own body's natural urges, which can lengthen the pushing phase overall. It can also have the potential to indeed cause swelling of her cervix, or cause the baby's head to end up with diffused swelling, called 'caput succedaneum'. If you feel that there are too many questions being asked of her regarding what she is feeling, then you can either chat to the midwife about trying not to 'overanalyse' this stage, or perhaps you would prefer to whisper into the woman's ear an agreed mantra, such as 'follow your body' or 'be guided by your body's own natural sensations'. Perhaps remind her that her baby's head needs time to mold to the space in her pelvis, and there is no rush for this to happen. This should hopefully prompt her to remember that there is no pressure to perform, and she should wait in this instance until the 'couldn't stop it if you tried' pushing kicks in.

Technique

I don't usually direct a woman on how to push, but there are a few things I like to alert her to in advance.

- **Sound**. All her sounds should go DOWNWARDS! There is no point in screaming out your baby; it is just not helpful. When sounds go up and out through the shoulders and head, they are wasting energy that should be directed down to where the energy needs to go. A woman with an instinctual urge is unlikely to scream, but if the woman you are supporting does, then help her to direct her efforts downwards by making low vibrational sounds with her like 'oh' or 'ahh' or 'maa'.
- **Hands**. Many women like to grip onto something when they are pushing. I often see their arms rise as the baby moves lower, and I offer my hands or clothing for her to squeeze (see Figure 6.5).

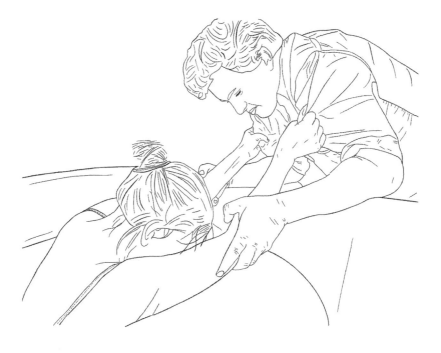

Figure 6.5

- **Relaxation**. Other women like to soften and relax every muscle in their body while they are pushing, preferring not to clench everything as in the example above.

- **Position**. Women may need to change their position a few times during this stage of labour. She may instinctively want to open her pelvis more, or she may want to stand or kneel. Sometimes it takes a walk up the stairs or a trip to the loo to help a baby round a certain part of the pelvis.

- **Releasing fears**. Every now and again I think I am seeing the woman hold back. It is not always easy to tell, but if I think it might be happening, I will ask her between surges to tell me what is on her mind. Sometimes she will be quick to respond and might shout out words like 'I'm scared of tearing', or 'I'm frightened I won't be a good mother'. Helping her to verbalise and then release these thoughts can make a huge difference to her pelvic floor muscles, which may have been pulled tight with all the fear she is holding onto.

- **'Reversing the chi'**. Another trick I have used in labour is something called 'reversing the chi'. It can be effective in the event that the woman feels the baby is 'stuck'. It is achieved by actively encouraging her not to push for three contractions. Instead, she needs to physically draw the baby upwards, like she is sucking it up and into her ribcage. After three full contractions, she should then go back to doing whatever her body is telling her.

'I Need to Push' vs Actual Pushing

If the woman you are supporting shares with you that she is 'feeling an urge to push', then usually this is an obvious sign that she definitely isn't quite ready to begin pushing. She may be describing a sensation that she is experiencing during her contraction, often at the peak. It's the same as if she is feeling the urge to go to the toilet, but not actually pooing. Sometimes at this stage, a woman can fall asleep between the longer gaps between contractions, which again is a clear sign that her body is working hard but not quite awake enough for the expulsive pushes that will soon follow. Try not to get excited by the words 'I need to push'. You are trying to avoid a situation where a woman who thinks she is close begins to push because she is impatient and believes the feeling of an urge is a clear sign that she is ready. Sometimes the position of the baby's head may trigger a sensation prematurely, which may explain why she is feeling like the urge is there. You can of course remind her that the sensations are normal if you think it would be helpful for her to hear this, but that she shouldn't push if she has to actively use any effort. I recommend you talk to her antenatally about how important it is for her to follow her body. You can ensure she understands the difference between feeling an urge to push, versus the sensation of being-unable-to-stop-it-if-she-tried actual pushing.

IMPORTANT TO KNOW *On the day, you should see that, at some stage, the pressure will move from her belly to her rectum, and active pushing will begin with a feeling of needing to bear down. At this point, she won't have to tell you that she feels an urge, because you will hear it and see it for yourself.*

Purple Pushing

Valsalva pushing, otherwise known as 'purple pushing', has been common practice for decades. With the rise in epidurals and assisted birth, it became the cultural norm for a woman to be told how and when to push. The woman is directed by her midwife or doctor to put her chin on her chest and 'push push push' into her bottom whilst holding her breath. In the UK it is fair to say that most midwives understand that this is not beneficial to mother or baby, as it restricts oxygen to the baby whilst the mother is being encouraged to hold her breath for long periods of time, far longer than she might normally do instinctively. This is something that she can request to avoid on her birth plan, and I would highly recommend she does so.

Don't Push with Her

I have to admit, this is not easy. I have on many occasions been aware that I was pushing at the same time as a client. If she doesn't know you are doing it, then obviously that's ok, but do try not to coach her in any way, or get involved with holding your own breath as she is pushing, as it can also look like you are guiding her. A woman who holds her own breath for as long as she wants to will never do any harm as it is usually only for short natural spells.

Where There is Poop, a Baby's Head Is Not Far Behind

Most women will empty their bowels either before labour or during the early stages. This is helpful because later on the baby will press on the rectum as it comes down, causing whatever may still be inside to be squeezed out. Usually there is very little left by the pushing stage; however, if she does poo, the midwives are incredibly discreet at clearing this away, so you as the birth partner may have no idea. My advice is to always expect it, and always ignore it. It is part of the process of birth and is a promising sign that the baby will be born soon.

She Won't Have the Energy to Push!

Over the years, I have heard it said to women many times that because she is so exhausted, she won't have the energy to push out her baby when the time comes. This statement is often used as a way to promote an intervention that the woman is not keen to accept. As the birth partner, you should know that if she is unmedicated and she waits for her body's own impulses, she will always have 'the energy' because, like vomiting, she will simply have no choice in the matter. Encourage her to rest and relax and conserve her energy between every single contraction from the outset. Feed her regular snacks and sips of water as often as possible, and this should provide enough energy to continue in labour for as long as she wants to.

Back Birthers

Having written all that I have about the negative effects of a labouring woman lying on her back (see Chapter 8), every now and again I will be supporting a woman who right at the end switches round and lies on her back to push out her baby. She is often amazed afterwards, and shares with me that she thought giving birth on her back was considered bad. Whilst I teach avoidance of this position overall, I also truly believe that any position the woman instinctively chooses herself is never bad. It's the ones that are chosen for her that I encourage her to decline. There are four different shapes of pelvis (again, see Chapter 8), with variations of space from top to bottom, so it makes sense that some women will actually do fine birthing on their backs. In my experience with the women I have supported, they tend to adopt this position after the baby has passed through the curve of Carus (a particular curve in the birth canal) and is already on its way out. In this instance the hardest part is done and the baby is just waiting to be born.

Stretching and Stinging

Many women feel frustrated during the pushing phase, as they feel the baby moving forwards and backwards. The vaginal tissues are stretching gently and in their own time. At the point when the baby begins to 'crown' (the head is stretching the vaginal opening) the woman may feel a stinging or burning sensation, often described as the 'ring of fire'. This is an important warning to the woman to slow down her pushing, in order to guide her baby out slowly from this point. For most women, the stinging is short lived and is usually followed by a feeling of numbness.

IMPORTANT TO KNOW In my experience, if a woman is following her body and tunes into the stinging sensation, she is less likely to tear, as long as she is not tempted to push too forcefully. She can ask for the midwife to give her specific support in guiding the baby out slowly. You can help by remaining quiet so that she can hear any instructions being given by the midwife as the baby is born.

Epidural

If the woman you are supporting decides to have an epidural in labour, then she will not usually be able to feel her contractions and won't know when to push. Some women may feel a strong pressure in their bottom, which they will be able to work with, and others may allow their epidural to wear off slightly so that they can feel something in the background, but on the whole, they are going to need coaching. The problem is that the drugs used in the epidural have the power to paralyse the woman's lower body (see Figure 6.6), including her pelvic floor muscles, which are no longer able to guide the baby. The baby itself may be affected too, due to the use of Fentanyl (a morphine-like drug), which is included in the epidural and can make the baby sleepy—losing its way and struggling to get

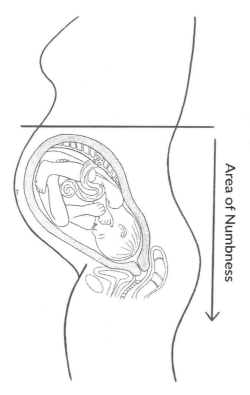

Area of Numbness

Figure 6.6

out. This means that the baby is four times more likely to remain in a persistently poor position, which decreases the woman's chances of a spontaneous birth. She will have no choice but to be directed to push and is also likely to be told to hold her breath for long periods. If you can get her into a comfortable side-lying position, and place a peanut-shaped ball or a stack of cushions between her top leg and her bottom leg (see Chapter 8) this will help the baby have more space to navigate, by creating as much room in the pelvis as possible. Once full dilation has been determined, the midwife usually leaves the mother alone for an hour or two, to encourage the baby to descend to a lower position. If the woman you are supporting would benefit from making more space in the pelvic outlet, you can encourage her to bring her knees together and widen her ankles away from her. This works best if the baby is already low.

Precipitous Birth

Occasionally a baby is born very quickly and catches everyone out with the labour's speed and intensity. Even though a fast birth may sound ideal to most, it can be shocking and incredibly traumatic to the woman, as her endorphins haven't had a chance to build, and she can often feel quite panicked by the experience. It might mean that you as the birth partner will have to 'catch' the baby if you are alone with her, or ideally you can encourage her to bring the baby up onto her chest herself. It depends on her position at the time. Unfortunately you cannot prevent a fast birth from happening, other than potentially encouraging her to put her bottom up in the air, to slow down the process if help is on it's way. If it appears that the birth you are attending is progressing quickly, then there are a few things that might help you to know.

- Stay calm and relaxed; a straightforward birth is usually nothing to worry about.
- Always try and call the community midwife to attend if you can, just in case they are able to help.

* If you call an ambulance, then try to ensure that the person on the end of the line doesn't take you away from the woman—for example to wait by the door, whereby you leave her on her own.

* Be sure to cover up the woman if she has no clothes on, and if both her and the baby are ok, let the paramedics know immediately so that they can arrive calmly rather than believing it is an emergency.

* If the baby has not been born by the time the paramedics arrive, don't automatically assume she has to travel to hospital if it is likely the baby will be born soon. In most cases it is safer to stay where you are rather than give birth in the ambulance on the way.

* Also, don't automatically assume you have to transfer to hospital after the baby is born if there is no medical reason to. You might be able to tuck mother and baby up in bed and stay where you are.

* Don't pacify the woman afterwards if she is struggling to cope with what happened to her. Tell her that you recognise how fast and shocking that was, and never describe what she went through as 'lucky'.

* Talk to her about seeking support if she needs to de-brief with a counsellor afterwards. Sometimes women describe feeling like they were going to die when a birth is so fast that they cannot process it, and PTSD (post-traumatic stress disorder) develops.

Unassisted Birth

In the UK, a small percentage of women will choose to give birth without a midwife or any other medical assistance present, known as unassisted birth or 'freebirth'. During the era of Covid-19, more and more women than ever chose to birth this way rather than leave their homes to go to hospital. As most home birth services were suspended during lockdown, these women felt they had no choice. In some cases, a woman will choose to give birth at home without a midwife because they have experienced a previous birth trauma, and want to avoid *any* potential medical interventions, not trusting the NHS to support them. If this is something that the woman you are supporting is considering, do your research and prepare well in advance. Doula Samantha Gadsden has a dedicated support group and has information on her website: **caerphillydoula.co.uk** (see the Resources section at the end of the book). In my experience, any woman choosing to freebirth will not make that decision lightly, so it is important to support her as much as you can. If you are seriously concerned and feel far out of your comfort zone, but she is confident in her decision, then perhaps look into hiring a doula that is willing to be with her alone, or with you both. It is perfectly legal in the UK for a woman to choose to give birth without a midwife present, as long as the people supporting her are not acting in the capacity of a midwife.

Vaginal Tears

After the birth, the midwife will want to check inside the woman's vagina to see if she has any grazes or tears. Sometimes, as the baby's head is born, the skin around the vaginal opening can be stretched too far, which can result in a tear of varying degrees.

The RCOG website categorises tears the following way:

- **First-degree:** Small tears affecting only the skin, which will heal without treatment
- **Second-degree:** Tears affecting the muscle of the perineum and the skin, which may require suturing (stitching together). These tears can be repaired by a midwife at home or in hospital. In some cases women may choose to let them heal naturally on their own and not have them sutured at all.
- **Third-** and **fourth-degree**: For 3.5% of women the tear is deeper and extends into the muscle that controls the anal sphincter. These tears will require repair in an operating theatre by a doctor.

For many women, the idea of tearing is more scary than the reality. The best way to avoid any tearing is to only push when she feels an overwhelming

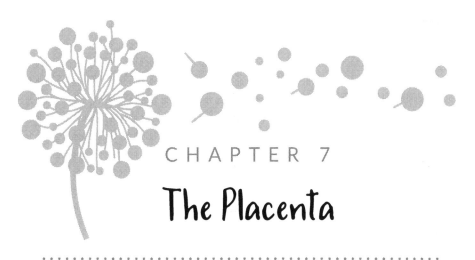

CHAPTER 7

The Placenta

We are the only species of mammal that doubts our ability to give birth. Think about that.

–Ina May Gaskin

After the baby is born, a woman's body and her hormones are working hard to ensure the final part of the birth process goes as smoothly as possible. Each woman needs a huge surge of oxytocin to reduce the adrenaline levels that were produced during the pushing stage. To help encourage this, make sure she is warm, covered up for privacy and ideally has skin-to-skin contact with the baby. Amongst the many benefits of the baby being skin to skin is the start of the bonding process, whilst at the same time, the baby's temperature, heart rate and breathing will begin to regularise. As time passes, and the mother's oxytocin levels rise, her uterine muscle fibres will begin to shorten, or retract, and she will start to feel contractions again. These lead to a gradual decrease in the size of the uterus, which helps to shear the placenta away from its attachment site on the mother's uterine wall.

Placenta Revolution

Over the past few years, I believe we have seen the start of a revolution when it comes to placentas. The role they play has become widely known

and identified as being beneficial for the baby, whereas previous genera-
tions thought it disgusting, called it the 'after birth' and had no desire to
even look at it. This new paradigm sees women recognising the brilliant
job that the placenta has done in growing their babies and keeping them
alive. In particular they are discovering that the placenta continues to
support the baby in those first vital minutes of the postnatal period, and
that it's important not to separate the baby from the placenta by cutting
the umbilical cord before its role is complete. Parents are learning and
understanding that in these early moments, the baby is transitioning, and
its lungs are beginning to inflate. At this time, the amount of blood left
in the placenta is approximately 30% of the baby's overall blood volume.
This blood belongs to the baby and is vital for growth and development.
In order to facilitate this process, the umbilical cord very cleverly begins
to pulsate, restricting the flow of blood going back to the placenta, and
quickly pumps the blood from the placenta into the baby. This miraculous
sequence of events takes place in the seconds and minutes that the baby is
learning to breathe for the first time, whilst still receiving lots of valuable
oxygen from the placenta. With the additional benefit of skin-to-skin contact from its mother, the process is gentle and kind for the baby.

The Umbilical Cord

The umbilical cord is cleverly designed, typically with three vessels—two
arteries and one vein—which transport blood, rich in oxygen and nutrients, to the baby and then return to the placenta with waste and carbon
dioxide. The cord is twisted, a bit like old telephone wire, and is filled with
a substance called Wharton's jelly. The jelly protects the vessels and is
responsible for helping the cord to keep its shape. The baby receives all
its oxygen through the umbilical cord, and the placenta acts as the lungs.
Even if the cord gets tied up in knots or wraps around the baby's neck like
a scarf or a full loop (known as a nuchal cord), its ability to function is
usually not affected. A nuchal cord is present in 20% to 30% of births, and

if a baby is born with the cord around its neck, the midwife will carefully slip the cord over the head as its body comes out. There should be no danger to the baby, unless the cord becomes compressed—which, whilst rare, can happen if the woman's waters break before the baby's head has engaged in the pelvis, and the cord slips down into the cervix (called cord prolapse). At the point of birth when the baby's lungs take over, the cord begins to pulsate, ensuring any remaining blood in the placenta will be pumped quickly into the baby. At the same time, the jelly inside the cord begins to liquefy, and the cord starts to unravel, going from very twisted, to loose and limp by the time it is empty (see Figure 7.1).

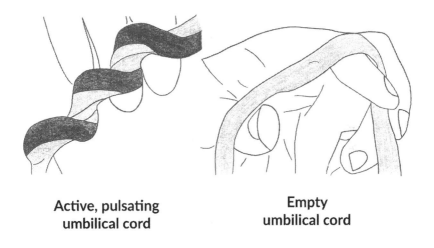

**Active, pulsating
umbilical cord**

**Empty
umbilical cord**

Figure 7.1

Clamping the Cord

Cutting and clamping the umbilical cord should not be at the forefront of anyone's mind in the immediate moments after birth, and the baby should be left alone so that its body can transition from womb to world gently. This is well documented as being in the best interests of the baby, and has been that way for centuries. Even as far back as 1801, Erasmus Darwin said

Another thing very injurious to the child, is the tying and cutting of the navel string too soon; which should always be left till the child has not only repeatedly breathed but till all pulsation in the cord ceases. As otherwise the child is much weaker than it ought to be, a portion of the blood being left in the placenta.

As birth moved to hospitals in the 1950s and 60s, however, and intervention rates began to climb, concerns about transference of anaesthetics and other drugs to the baby from the mother's blood led to immediate clamping and cutting of the cord. This was despite recommendations from experts and publications like The Lancet medical journal, which continued to clearly state that a clamp should not be used until the cord stopped pulsating and blood flow had ceased. To make matters worse, the midwife or doctor attending the woman would also feel for the umbilical cord around the baby's neck, and if it was discovered to be present, the cord was rapidly clamped and cut before the baby was even out, resulting in the baby's oxygen supply being cut off at an extremely crucial moment. As time went by, it became obvious that this was not best practice, it was not evidence-based, and it was dangerous to babies, so one or two brave midwives and doctors began to speak up.

Optimal Cord Clamping

Amanda Burleigh, a midwife from Leeds, became well known as an advocate for leaving the umbilical cord alone and preventing the issues that early clamping and cutting caused. She says on her website,

I started campaigning for optimal cord clamping in 2005. I had been qualified as a Midwife for 16 years, and after considerable reflection and researching of evidence, I spoke to primary school teachers who concurred that increasing numbers of children appeared to be suffering educational, behavioural and health problems. I reflected on our practice as clinicians and discovered that the routine practice of immediate (early/premature) cord clamping carried out after baby's birth but generally before the baby had taken its first breath was an intervention in natural physiology which had no evidence to support it.

When Dr. Alan Greene began speaking of optimal cord clamping in 2011 and outlined the TICC TOCC campaign during his TED talk in Brussels in 2012, he used the persuasive title '90 Seconds to Save the World'. You can watch it on his website, drgreene.com. He began with these words: 'Today we are going to talk about a very powerful idea that can transform the lives of children around the world. It's an idea that is simple, that is easy to implement, and costs nothing'. He shared that lack of oxygen at birth and lowered levels of iron because of immediate cord clamping was causing some babies to be affected for life. Simply leaving the cord alone would enable the third of the baby's blood volume that was outside of their body at the moment of birth to transfer. As the baby emerges, the umbilical cord begins to pulsate, pumping everything they need to thrive into them quickly and efficiently, as nature intended.

During this process, babies receive:

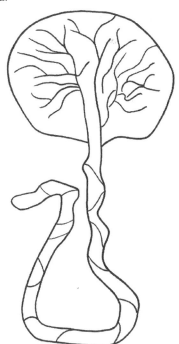

* 30% more iron-rich blood. It would take approximately 6 months to replenish this if lost at birth.
* More oxygen to the brain, which continues to be provided to them as their lungs transition.
* 60 % more red blood cells that carry oxygen, giving babies extra support.
* More white blood cells to help fight infections.
* More stem cells, which have the genetic potential to prevent and repair damage throughout the body.

#Wait for White

Amanda Burleigh was successful in helping to promote change within UK hospitals, and since 2014, the recommendation from NICE (National Institute for Health and Care Excellence) states that each baby born should be given at least one minute of time for their blood to transition. Unfortunately whilst this is great progress, she and many others feel that it would be far more optimal to leave the cord alone until it has stopped pulsating altogether. Her most recent campaign features the widely recognised slogan 'wait for white'. Only by leaving the cord alone until it has become white and empty can you ensure that all of the baby's blood has transferred, and optimal benefits have been received.

Requesting Optimal Cord Clamping

Leaving the cord alone to finish pulsating is a very personal preference and may not suit all women and their circumstances. For those that do request optimal cord clamping, it needs to be written clearly on their birth preferences, and, at the time of birth, repeated by the mother (or you as the birth partner). If a paediatrician is in the room, you should ensure they understand this is a strong preference and should be respected unless a dire emergency requires them to rush the baby to the special care baby unit (SCBU). In most cases, even if the baby requires some initial support to breathe, that can be done next to the mother with the cord intact, as it will continue to provide the baby with valuable oxygen.

Despite it being clearly specified on a woman's birth plan, the reality is that many midwives and doctors are still cutting the cord way too soon. If mum and baby are skin to skin and they are both well and comfortable, then there is absolutely no benefit to touching the cord at all. If, however, the woman is not comfortable or there is a reason why the baby needs to be moved, then a conversation can be had in that moment about whether the cord should be cut to separate the mother and baby. Sometimes a cord is short and may initially prevent the baby from being lifted onto the mother's chest; however, it should begin to lengthen as the cord unravels. You can see the change before your very eyes, and you have the option to physically touch the cord and feel it pulsate if you want to. As the cord lengthens and empties, it starts to become very obviously white and limp, so you will know when it is finished.

ANDY'S STORY Leanne and I had spoken in detail about leaving the cord to pulsate after the baby was born, so I knew it was important to her. As soon as our daughter was in Leanne's arms, the midwife was happy to leave us alone, where we spent about five minutes or more checking out her little fingers and toes, enjoying every moment. At some stage, I became aware that our midwife was back at our side, and as she caught my eye she asked me if I was 'ready to cut the cord'. I said yes and asked her if it was finished. 'Oh, yes', she replied, and began the process. At that point I looked down and said 'Wait, it's still looking quite active to me', and she confidently reassured me that it was fine and that baby had had all she needed as she secured the clamps in place. I have always felt that I let Leanne down in that moment, because I should have just asked her to give us more time. There was no benefit to cutting the cord, and I am cross that we did. We didn't move the baby, we didn't move Leanne, and the two remained together skin to skin for at least another 40 minutes or more. Next time I will be a lot more specific and will ask the midwife to wait.

Hormones

During the third stage of labour, it is important for the woman's oxytocin levels to rise once more. Signs that she is still filled with adrenaline in- clude: uncontrollable shaking, and being easily distracted by sounds and questions, instead of gazing into her baby's eyes. At this time, you can try to reduce the amount of adrenaline in her body as quickly as possible so that her oxytocin levels can pick up. This will really help with bonding and the birth of the placenta. I always go back to basics here and think about making her feel safe, warm, and loved. It is also important to check the environment where possible to make sure she has privacy, darkness and quiet.

IMPORTANT TO KNOW   *Not all women will want to hold the baby immediately, as some need a bit of time to gather themselves after the birth. If you are her spouse, or family member, then you can place the baby skin to skin on your own chest until she is ready.*

The Golden Hour

The period of time after a baby is born should be unhurried. Ideally, the baby will not be touched by anyone other than the parents, where possible, for at least an hour. As the baby lies on its mother's chest, a series of important events start to happen. The baby's temperature begins to regulate, as the mother is designed to be a human incubator: quite cleverly, if the baby cools down, the mother will warm up, and vice versa. At the same time, the body becomes colonised with bacteria from the mother's skin and mouth as she touches and kisses the baby. This is vital to building a healthy immune system and helps prevent allergic responses. Mothers who choose to establish breastfeeding may find that the golden hour is a nice relaxed time for this to begin (see Chapter 16). Often the baby will find its own way to the breast if given time and patience. Skin-to-skin contact with the baby during the golden hour also enables important hormones to be released that are crucial for the bonding process. In some hospitals and MLUs, the midwife will actually place a large egg timer in the room to remind the staff to leave the baby alone so that it can remain skin to skin with its mother. This means they are not allowed to touch, move or weigh the baby during this time. Milli Hill, founder of the Positive Birth Movement and author of *The Positive Birth Book,* calls this 'The Hour of Power'. I recommend that, as the birth partner, you do your best to use the PROTECTS tool as outlined in Chapter 9. During this time, make sure that the mother and baby are in a comfortable position, that the mother has something to eat and drink, and that the environment facilitates this special time, with no pressure to do or think of anything else. If it is obvious that the golden hour cannot start immediately, then as soon as it is possible, ensure that everyone is aware that you want to help the mother and baby re-create this, and that she would like skin to skin with no interruptions. In neonatal units across the world this is called 'kangaroo care', and is widely promoted to help improve outcomes for premature babies.

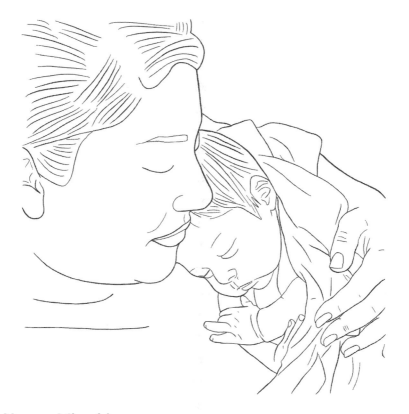

Human Microbiome

During the birth process, microbes are passed on to the baby that are essential for building the immune system. Vital bacteria such as lactobacilli head to the vagina in preparation for birth, and as the baby passes through, bacteria begin to colonise the baby's intestinal tract and helps to 'seed' the baby's gut.

The baby receives microbes from the:

- Placenta
- Umbilical cord
- Amniotic fluid
- Mother's vagina
- Parents' skin
- Parents' mouth
- Breast milk
- Siblings and pets

A healthy immune system is developed when the baby is exposed to bacteria from all of the above, and what could be better than the germs of its own parents to begin the process, and not others in the birth room. This includes any birth partner who is not directly related to the baby—I personally never touch a newborn baby when working in the role of a doula. The thousands of different organisms within us are essential to keeping the baby safe, as 70% of our immune system is located in the gut. This makes skin-to-skin contact even more important for at least an hour after birth, although she can of course continue for as long as she wants to.

IMPORTANT TO KNOW   *At the point when it is time to weigh the baby, I would encourage you to carry the baby to and from the scales yourself. This helps by preserving the newborn microbiome as much as possible.*

Antibiotics

Approximately 30% of babies, although it varies from hospital to hospital, are born via caesarean section in the UK each year. During surgery, the mother is given antibiotics, which the baby is then exposed to via the placenta and colostrum. In addition, as the baby is not exposed to the bacteria in the birth canal, and does not go straight to its mother, it is more likely to be colonised by hospital bacteria in the early moments of birth. In this instance, the parents should do their best to help colonise the baby's gut with their own bacteria as quickly as possible, and both the mother and baby should replenish the friendly bacteria wiped out by the antibiotics.

For this reason, I recommend that all parents do the following: Sleep with some blankets or muslin cloth, (three or four) during pregnancy, and if there are other kids or pets at home, then they should be exposed to the blankets too. I'm not suggesting that they are dragged around the floor or anything, but they should be slept with and drooled on, and coated with as much bacteria from home as possible, from the skin and mouths of the parents and siblings. On the day of the birth, place them in a clean bag and have them easily accessible. If the baby has to be removed from the mother in the instance that they are unwell, or a c-section is performed, the muslin cloth or blanket can be placed in direct contact with the baby, between the baby's skin and the hospital towel that will be used to wrap the baby in.

You can then purchase a high quality probiotic—both a paediatric one for the newborn and an extra strength one for the mother. These can be bought online or from a knowledgeable health food store that stocks both. BioCare, Optibac and BioGaia are the brands my clients use most.

If you are curious to find out more about how important the microbiome is to a newborn baby, watch the amazing film "Microbirth" made by Toni Harman and Alex Wakeford. Released in 2014, this incredible documentary investigates the latest scientific research on the microscopic events happening during childbirth. These events can have serious implications for the lifelong health of children.

An imbalance in the microbiome can contribute to:

* Eczema
* Acne
* Asthma
* Allergies
* Diabetes

- Coeliac
- IBS
- Mental health issues
- Chronic fatigue
- Parkinson's disease
- MS and other immune system diseases

In the early days of a baby's life, the more common results of such an imbalance are thrush, skin issues and sleep problems.

IMPORTANT TO KNOW   *This is the same for babies who are born vaginally but given antibiotics postnatally for health concerns or a suspected infection.*

Physiological vs Managed Third Stage

The third stage (the name commonly given to this time) is complete when the mother births her baby's placenta. There are two options available:

1. The first, called a physiological third stage, is where the placenta can be left to come out on its own.

2. The second is where the woman can be given an oxytocic injection and the placenta can be guided out by the midwife.

If the woman you are supporting is undecided which option to choose, she doesn't need to make a decision until the baby is born.

Physiological Third Stage

If the woman you are supporting has decided that she would like a physiological third stage, then you can expect that after having skin-to-skin contact with the baby for a while, she may start to feel noticeable contractions again. Whilst they are a lot less intense than the ones felt in the final stages of labour, they can still be very uncomfortable for her. This happens as her oxytocin levels begin to rise, and can be more noticeable if the baby is breastfeeding. As the uterus shrinks, the placenta will peel away and the woman can often, with a gentle push, help to ease it out. It is common to see a gush of blood (up to 500 ml is considered normal) at this point. The length of time between the birth of the baby and the placenta separating from the uterine wall can typically range from a few minutes to, in some cases, an hour or more. Once out, the midwife will catch the placenta in a bowl and take it away to examine, making sure that it is complete and that no part of it has remained inside the uterus.

If the birth was a shock in any way, or there are too many people around, the woman can struggle to lower her adrenaline levels, causing the placenta to be slow to separate. In this instance, I recommend checking to see if privacy might be causing an issue, so consider the following questions.

- Are there too many people around?
- Is the room too bright?
- Is she warm enough?
- Does she feel under pressure to begin breastfeeding?
- Is she being asked too many questions?

IMPORTANT TO KNOW *If you suspect a 'yes' answer to any of these questions, try to get her into the bathroom, put her on the toilet, wrap her in a big blanket and close the door. If she is able to empty her bladder, have some quiet and privacy, it can usually help raise her oxytocin levels and the placenta comes away.*

Blood Loss

You would expect a woman to lose blood and blood clots at this stage, so don't be too shocked if she is bleeding what may appear to you as heavily. Anything up to 500 ml (a pint) is considered normal. The midwife will want to visually measure how much, and if blood loss is deemed to be high, may recommend a managed third stage, using an oxytocin injection to help stem the blood loss.

Managed Third Stage

The option of an oxytocin injection to help the uterus contract is available at any point after birth. The mixture of oxytocin and ergometrine can be very helpful in reducing heavy blood loss, so it may be offered in the event that the midwife or doctor are worried that the woman is bleeding heavily. If a woman had a long labour that resulted in high levels of intervention, it may also be strongly recommended. Some women may choose to have this injection administered immediately, and others may wait and have it later if there is still no sign of the placenta. Once the injection is given, the midwife will need to pull on the umbilical cord as it begins to separate from the uterine wall. This is called 'controlled cord traction'. The midwife needs to help the placenta out before the uterus and cervix closes with the placenta left inside (known as retained placenta). The benefits of having the injection include getting the placenta out quickly and helping to reduce heavy blood loss by narrowing the blood vessel walls. Risks include increased blood pressure, nausea and vomiting, plus the potential for a retained placenta which would involve the woman being taken to theatre for it to be removed manually under anaesthetic.

Cutting the Cord

When it is time to cut the umbilical cord, the midwife will place a plastic clamp near to the baby's belly button, and after leaving a gap, will place a scissor-like clamp on the other side. One or both of the parents are usually invited to cut between the two clamps; however this is completely optional, and if the parents decline the midwife will do it. As many families are choosing to avoid the use of plastic when possible, ask the woman you are supporting if she is happy to use the standard plastic clamps provided by the hospital, or alternatively, she can provide her own umbilical cord tie, made from embroidery thread, which can be homemade or purchased online.

Lotus Birth

Some families might choose not to cut the cord at all, but to leave the placenta attached to the baby. This is believed to be a much more gentle transition, and it is thought that the baby will be calmer and more peaceful overall. It is a practice that honours the connection between the baby and its placenta as a vital organ that has provided nourishment beautifully in the womb. It is therefore up to the baby when that connection is severed, with the cord falling off in its own time. During the early stage of the process, the woman and her family will need to treat the placenta with certain ingredients to maintain its freshness, and choose a bag to carry the placenta in. There is lots of support out there for anyone who chooses this option. Check the website **babyprepping.com** and the Resources section at the end of this book.

Placenta Encapsulation

Placenta encapsulation is a process where a woman's placenta is transformed into pills that she will consume daily in the early postnatal period. In recent years it has become very popular, and there are trained specialists all over the world. The placenta will need to be chilled within 30 minutes after the birth, and then collected by a specialist who takes it away to dry it out, grind it down and encapsulate it into pills that the mother will swallow. The anecdotal evidence for this service is incredible, with benefits including:

* Increased energy levels
* Greater milk supply
* Reduced blood loss
* Reduced likelihood of postnatal depression

I personally have yet to meet a woman who hasn't loved the way her placenta pills made her feel in the postnatal period. If this is something that the woman you are supporting is interested in, then I recommend you look into which specialists cover your area. The person hired to encapsulate will provide you with specific instructions that you should read in advance of labour starting. You should also make yourself aware of what equipment is required, as the placenta will need to be chilled very quickly, and this task usually falls to the birth partner.

QUICK RECAP

Here are the main things to remember when discussing the placenta.

- **The importance of the placenta's role.** The placenta is a major organ that is connected to the baby via the umbilical cord. It plays a very important role in the baby's growth and acts as its lungs, liver, gut and kidneys.

- **The umbilical cord will begin to pulsate.** Approximately 30% of the baby's blood volume is within the placenta at the moment of birth, and as long as the umbilical cord remains intact, the cord will begin to pulsate and quickly transfer the blood into the baby.

- **Increase oxytocin levels.** The mother's oxytocin levels will need to rise for the uterus to begin to shrink down so the placenta can separate from it. Keep her warm and cover her for extra privacy at this time.

- **The importance of skin to skin.** The mother can enjoy the benefits of having the baby skin to skin, which supports them both during the transition from womb to world. As vital hormones are being released to establish bonding, the baby's temperature, breathing and heartrate are also becoming established.

- **The uterus closes down.** The woman may feel strong contractions as her uterus closes down, which can increase in intensity the more children she has.

- **Managed third stage.** If she would like, she can have an injection of the synthetic form of oxytocin to help speed up the placenta separating from the uterine wall. This can help with blood loss.

CHAPTER 8

Positions

It is important to keep in mind that our bodies must work pretty well, or there wouldn't be so many humans on the planet.

-Ina May Gaskin

The distance a baby has to travel on the day it is born is not that far at all, yet it is still quite a journey. Just a few centimeters can take many hours, and the woman's mobility and position during that time is critical in facilitating the process. If she is able to learn and practice positions during pregnancy, it will help her know exactly how to maximise the space she has in her pelvis. She should begin with daily stretches that help her relax and release tense muscles and ligaments. It is also beneficial to have a really good understanding of how the baby moves through the pelvis and what positions make this easier. Helping the baby adopt a particular position in pregnancy is not essential; however, it is often thought to be optimal if the baby has its spine toward the front (anterior) of the mothers' body. During labour, there are lots of positions she can adopt to maximise space for the baby, creating more room to move around, which I will share with you in this chapter. All of these positions are ones that I practise with my clients regularly, and they can all be used in a variety of locations.

The Female Pelvis

The female pelvis, which is wider than that of the male, comes in a variety of structural shapes. In medical school, doctors and midwives are taught about the four most widely recognised shapes. Of those, over 50% of Caucasian women have a Gynecoid pelvis, while nearly half of women of African descent have an Anthropoid shape. About 25% of all women have an Android pelvis, and only 5% are said to have a Platypelloid pelvis (see Figure 8.1). During pregnancy, the hormone relaxin enables the pelvis to become more mobile, softening the ligaments and joints in preparation for the baby to pass through. As labour begins, and the baby moves down, regardless of what shape pelvis the woman has, the soft bones in the baby's head will mould to fit the space.

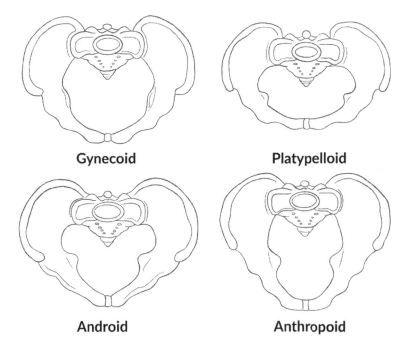

Gynecoid	**Platypelloid**
Android	**Anthropoid**

Figure 8.1 Variations of the female pelvis

At the top of the pelvis (known as the brim or inlet) where the baby first begins to descend, it is widest from left to right or hip to hip. Once the baby's head is in the pelvic cavity (or mid-pelvis), it needs to rotate around in order for the shoulders to have enough room to drop in. This lines up the head with the outlet, which is widest from front to back. The baby will usually then turn again to birth the shoulders, like a key turning in a lock (see Figure 8.2). It's helpful if the woman can adopt an upright or side-lying position during this time, because her sacrum (triangular bone at the base of the spine) and coccyx (tailbone) then have the ability to lift and move out of the way. This enables the pelvis to open up by as much as 30%, creating even more space for the baby to pass through.

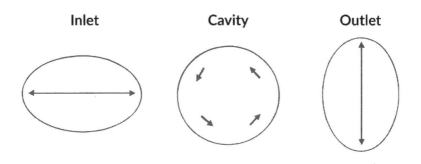

Figure 8.2 The baby needs to rotate in the pelvic cavity as it is being born.

Positions in Early Labour

Whilst gravity is helpful to dilate the cervix, it is also important that a woman in labour rests as much as possible, especially in the early stages, in order to conserve her energy for what is to follow. In some cases, women can be awake for at least one or two consecutive nights when giving birth, so it's best to plan for the long haul.

It is the job of the birth partner to remind her of the following:

- As soon as labour begins, rest.
- As labour picks up, rest.
- Between sensations, rest.
- If labour slows, rest.

I recommend that if labour starts at night, the woman remains in bed for as long as possible, so that she can sleep between contractions. If you are with her at this stage, stay out of her eyeline as much as you can, so that she doesn't feel overly observed or distracted. I really recommend you sleep too, as you won't have the ability to keep supporting her if you are exhausted. If labour begins in the daytime, she can move around and experiment with any position she finds the most comfortable, as long as she is relaxing and not doing too much. I often hear of women who bounce vigorously on their ball, clean the house, or go on long walks. In my experience, these are the women who share postnatally that they wished they had rested as they hadn't anticipated how exhausted they would feel during and after the birth.

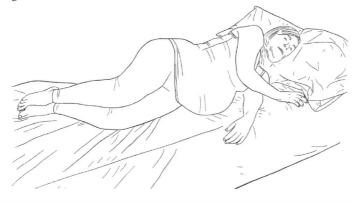

Resting between contractions during early labour will conserve energy and help the woman relax as much as possible.

If the contractions are too intense for her to continue to lie down during each one, then she can roll off the sofa into an all-fours position on her hands and knees, which will enable her to rock and move her hips if she wants to. This position also takes the weight of the baby off her spine, which makes it more comfortable for her during each surge.

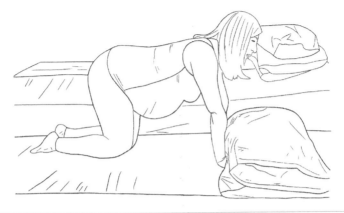

An all-fours position helps her mobilise during a contraction. She can then go back to lying down and resting in between.

Upright Forward and Open

If she prefers to adopt more upright positions, the following should help in early labour.

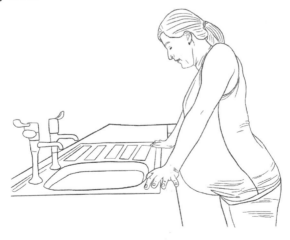

Leaning against a kitchen work top, or piece of furniture that gives good support like the back of a chair or sofa, can work well if she wants her feet grounded on the floor and she is comfortable standing upright.

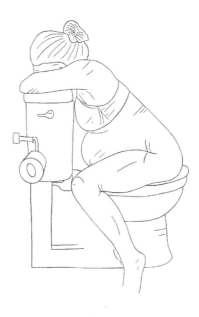

Straddling the toilet or a chair will open the pelvis and offer support for her to rest while leaning forward.

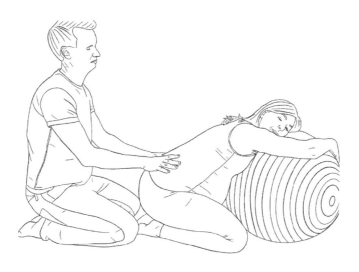

She can lean over a ball or pile of cushions whilst the birth partner offers to massage her or puts pressure on her lower back, if needed.

Relaxing All Muscles

As the labour intensifies, you should pay particular attention to her shoulders and her jaw. These are key areas for holding tension, and she should be encouraged to relax and soften if you notice that she is struggling to let go. Practicing hypnobirthing skills with her in pregnancy will really help (see Chapter 11), including simple stroking techniques and anchor words.

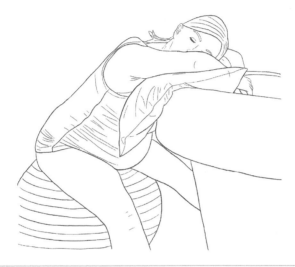

Sitting on a birth ball and leaning over the edge of the sofa, chair, table or pool with her head resting on a cushion is helpful between contractions. If she likes to stand up whilst having a contraction, it is then easy for her to sit and return to her rest position in between, relaxing and softening her muscles once more.

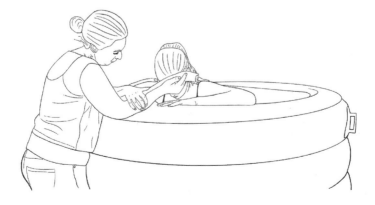

She can lean over the edge of the birth pool, resting on a cold flannel.

If All You Have Is a Bed

If you are in a hospital, and all that is available to you is a bed, then there are many different ways to be creative.

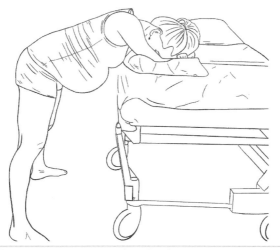

Raise the bed up as high as you want to by using the control panel at the side of the bed. Get it to exactly the right height so she can lean over and relax.

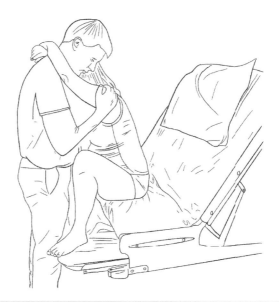

Make the hospital bed into a chair by lowering the bottom and raising the back upright.

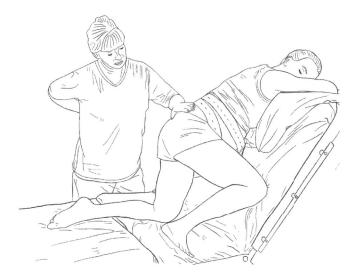

The mattress on the bed can be more comfortable and softer under her knees. If she wants to get on the bed, encourage her to lean forward. You can raise the back of the bed if you need to.

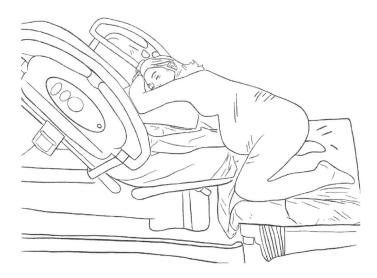

Alternatively, you can lower the bottom section of the bed as well as raising the back. This helps her get comfortable by enabling her to lean forward. Some women may like to use extra pillows under her head and perhaps also underneath her bum for greater support.

Keep Her Off Her Back

No matter what equipment you have to hand, there are many ways to keep a labouring woman off her back in order to maximise room in the pelvis. Be inventive and take cushions with you to the hospital or beg, borrow and steal them from the midwife. In the event of her being continuously monitored, or if she decides to have an epidural, you can lie her on her side and raise her leg up to a comfortable level using the cushions or a peanut-shaped birth ball. This opens the pelvis as much as possible and keeps the baby in a position that may facilitate a smooth and easier birth.

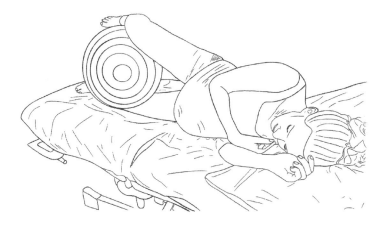

Lying on her side with a peanut ball or cushions between her legs can open up her pelvis to create more space for the baby to move down while the woman you are supporting gets a rest. This is useful for any stage of labour.

> The mum's job is to dilate and the baby's job is to rotate; being head down is not enough.
>
> –Gail Tully, founder of Spinning Babies

The Rhombus de Michaelis

During the process of pushing the baby out, the triangular bone at the base of the woman's spine (sacrum) has the capability to move, and her lower back will lift, opening up to create more space. The sacrum is within this kite shaped area just below her waist and is called 'The Rhombus de Michaelis' (see Figure 8.3). At this time, if the baby still needs to turn, it will be essential to maximise the extra space required, so a good upright and forward position is important to facilitate descent and rotation of the baby. When a woman is pushing, you might see her lift her arms upwards in order to feel more stable and secure.

IMPORTANT TO KNOW   *Helping to support a woman through this stage can be very physical at times, and in the event that progress is slow, just remember that the more space she can create, the better.*

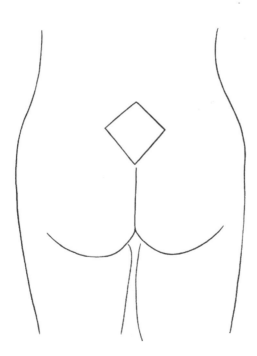

Figure 8.3 Rhombus de Michaelis

Back to Back

Sometimes a baby turns in pregnancy or during labour into a position known as OP (occiput posterior) or 'back to back'. An OP position occurs when the baby's spine is towards its mother's spine. If the baby struggles to rotate during labour, this can be the cause of a delay. Between 15% and 30% of babies start labour in an OP position, but fewer than 5% will remain in this position at birth. Anything that you change in the physiological process of birth is an intervention, but in this instance, you might want to have a look at the Spinning Babies website (**spinningbabies.com**). On the website there are suggestions of positions that can be beneficial in encouraging the baby to turn so that its spine is facing towards the front.

IMPORTANT TO KNOW *If the woman is describing feeling her contractions as being more in her back, then you can try using firm pressure on her sacrum during each contraction, to bring her some relief.*

Pelvic Girdle Pain

Pelvic girdle pain (PGP) is the name given to any pain felt in and around the pelvis, which includes the symphysis pubis joint at the front and sacroiliac joints at the back. The pelvic partnership website pelvicpartnership.org.uk says ' PGP is a biomechanical pelvic joint problem, previously known as Symphysis Pubis Dysfunction (SPD). PGP affects 1 in 5 pregnant women and symptoms can occur at any stage during or following pregnancy. PGP causes pain and stiffness in the pelvic joints, and difficulty walking, climbing stairs and turning in bed.' If a woman is experiencing any form of PGP, I recommend she see a specialist, which may include Bowen, Osteopathy, Chiropractic or Physiotherapy professionals. This may help to stabilise the pelvis, which can offer relief. During labour, it is important for the woman not to open her knees too wide, as this can be very painful. Upright positions, standing or leaning forward are all suitable. Most women with PGP love to give birth in water as this gives them the ability to keep their knees together and they can move around easily.

Knees Together

During the pushing stage, some babies benefit from extra room being created in the pelvic outlet, which can be achieved by the woman bringing her knees in closer together and pushing the ankles and feet apart. This is particularly helpful if the baby is visible by the midwives, but not moving down. If the woman is upright and leaning forward, this is easy to achieve by simply moving her ankles away from her. If she is lying on her side, perhaps with an epidural in place, then I recommend using a peanut-shaped ball or a big pile of cushions to prop her feet apart whilst dropping her knees together.

IMPORTANT TO KNOW *Practice this position during the pregnancy so that you both know how to achieve a knees-together position. Look at what happens when she splays her feet out wide and away from her knees. Notice how the lowest part of her pelvis (the outlet) can open wider.*

Shoulder Dystocia

Many women are told during pregnancy that their pelvis is small or that their baby is big, and that the baby has the potential to become 'stuck' on the way out. The doctor or midwife may talk of 'shoulder dystocia' which is where one of the baby's shoulders can catch on the mother's pelvic bone during the birth. As you can imagine, this causes anxiety in many women and leaves a lasting fear in their minds around the success of a safe vaginal birth. In fact, shoulder dystocia occurs in about 1 in 150 (0.7%) vaginal births, which makes it incredibly unlikely and, in my opinion, that number would be reduced further if there were fewer women lying on their backs to give birth. If the woman you are supporting is thought to be carrying a large baby, she may be offered the opportunity to attend a growth scan appointment, which she can choose to accept or decline. If she is happy to accept then it is important that she understands the scan will not be able to predict whether this might happen to her baby during labour, regardless of size, and half of all instances of shoulder dystocia occur in babies weighing less than 9 lbs (about 4 kg).

IMPORTANT TO KNOW *The Royal College of Obstetricians and Gynaecologists (RCOG) state that ultrasound scans are not good at telling whether you are likely to have a large baby and therefore they are not recommended for predicting shoulder dystocia, if you have no other risk factors.*

Whilst it is impossible to predict when shoulder dystocia will happen, it is more likely to take place if the woman:

- Had this occur in a previous pregnancy.
- Has diabetes.
- Has a high body mass index (BMI).
- Has her labour induced.
- Has a long labour.
- Has an assisted vaginal birth (forceps or ventouse).

QUICK RECAP

Here are the main things to remember when discussing positions.

- **Create more space in the pelvis.** The pelvic inlet is widest at the top from side to side. In early labour, a position where the woman is leaning forward with her knees wide apart, can create plenty of space for the baby to drop down.
- **Practice positions.** Look closely at the examples of different positions for early labour and practice them together in pregnancy. She will most likely show a preference for some more than others.

- **Rest between contractions.** Encourage her to rest and 'flop' between contractions to enable her mind and body to relax as much as possible.
- **Empty the bladder.** Regular visits to the toilet will help get her to move every hour or two and to open up the pelvis as she sits down. Encourage her to stay there for as long as she can, and close the door so she gets some privacy.
- **Adjust during the pushing stage.** If she has been pushing for some time, and the baby is slow to be born, remember that the pelvic outlet is widest from front to back. If the baby is low, she can bring her knees closer together and her ankles wider apart, which creates more space. Practice this in pregnancy too.

CHAPTER 9

The Birth Partner

If a woman doesn't look like a goddess during labour, then someone isn't treating her right.

–Ina May Gaskin

Whilst this whole book focuses on the role of the birth partner, there are some specific things I wanted to share with you that don't fit into any of the other chapters: things like how it feels to be on call, what practical elements you're 'in charge' of on the day, and what a doula—professional birth partner—is. Let's start there.

Doulas

Simply by reading this book, you no doubt take your role as a birth partner very seriously. Whilst the information covered in the chapters is designed to prepare you for that job, you might still be unsure of how you are going to cope. This is perfectly normal, and it's ok to admit that the responsibility of being a birth partner feels pretty overwhelming. It is fair to say that not all life partners, relatives or friends make good birth partners, and many of you reading this will recognise that lack of experience is probably not ideal when it comes to having a baby. An extra pair of hands that belong to someone who is confident, trained and experienced in coping with pregnancy and preparing for childbirth is fast becoming one of the most important tools in any couple's toolbox.

Imagine you were planning a trip to the Himalayas. In your mind, you will climb the tallest peaks, and after a long and tiring journey, you will be rewarded by reaching the highest summits, to stand on top of the world in awe of the incredible views. Now imagine turning around to see your Sherpa beside you. Whilst you may have planned this journey for many years, read the books and trained to the peak of physical fitness, you recognise the need for an experienced person who knows the area, has been there many times before, and speaks the native language. Travelling without them is unthinkable.

A 'doula' (a Greek word meaning caregiver), is just like that Sherpa! They help women and their partners throughout pregnancy, birth and the early postnatal period, ensuring that they have a positive experience overall by providing emotional, physical and educational support. Many couples who hire a doula recognise the value of an experienced guide, and rather than see a doula as someone who replaces the spouse or family member in the birth room, they understand that a doula can enhance others' roles. By working as part of a team, the birth partner will also feel confident, well supported and more able to offer love to the labouring woman, which in turn will raise her oxytocin levels.

A doula:

- Is a familiar face whom the couple grow to trust.
- Has no emotional connection to the woman (unlike a mother, sister, or best friend).
- Helps the woman to achieve her preferences.
- Bridges the gap among busy medical professionals by being a constant presence.
- Provides support to the birth partner in addition to the pregnant woman.

- Advocates, where necessary, by providing the couple with educational information, helping them to make well informed decisions.

The presence of a calm, confident, encouraging person, who understands the woman's physiological needs and knows her preferences and how to achieve them, can literally make all the difference to the labouring woman and her birth partner. An experienced doula can confidently see what is happening in any given moment, stepping up support when required and stepping back when not. This is an important element of the role, in my opinion, in order to avoid too much 'coaching' from different sources. With my clients, I like to explain that if all is going well, and the midwife and woman are establishing a good bond, I will reduce my vocal guidance and enable their relationship to develop, but be there for her offering physical support if needed. I describe this to my clients as 'reading the room', helping her to recognise that she does not need to have too many people surround her at one time.

Cost

As this service is predominantly private (although there are some areas of the UK that provide free doula support to vulnerable women), it does come at a cost. At the time of writing this book in 2020, the average cost of a doula in the UK is approximately £1,500 for a basic birth package, with many doulas charging higher rates in the south of England, and lower in the north. It is easy to find doulas in your area simply by googling the question 'doula in my area' or 'doula in (town name)'. There are plenty of doula directories, and you can also look at the Doula UK website, **doula.org.uk**, and use the 'find a doula' search engine, which will show you doulas who are local to you within the range that you request. As well as experienced, or 'recognised', doulas, the Doula UK website lists 'mentored' doulas who are still in the first year or two of their practice. These doulas can often be a little cheaper, as you will be required to evaluate them and provide feedback to their mentor.

Can We Afford to Hire a Doula?

Hiring a doula is described as an absolute necessity by my clients, and a typical comment that I hear isn't 'Can we afford to?'; it's 'Can we afford not to?' Whilst preparing for a blog a few years ago, I asked an online group some questions about what they considered the most important days of their life. It was no surprise to find out that everyone who replied (several hundred) said it was the day of their wedding (those that were married) and the day that their child or children were born. When I asked what they had spent on the cost of their wedding, the range was between £10,000 and £30,000. When I asked them what they spent on their birth, they all said £0. Many acknowledged during the online discussion, that they would have benefitted from doula support. Some shared that the negative effects of their birth experience were ongoing, and some couples admitted that they were not going to have any more children because of how their first birth had played out. One couple, having initially thought it was too expensive, admitted that in hindsight, they wished they had researched further. They felt they would have truly benefited from doula support, which they worked out would have cost less than their daily visit to Starbucks for a year. They have now started to save for their next baby. No one can dispute the fact that the memories of giving birth last a lifetime; if you ever sit down and speak to a 75-year-old woman about her birth experience 40 to 50 years earlier, she will be able to remember every detail, and specifically how she felt and how she was treated.

Obviously I believe that every woman and her birth partner should hire a doula for their birth. I know, however, that it is not possible for all families, for a variety of reasons, not to mention that there are not enough of us to go round. For this reason, I am hoping that each one of the chapters in this book will help you understand how important you are to the birth process, and to make sure that even if you have never done this before, you can become familiar with the landscape and learn to speak some of the native language, just like the Sherpas.

> A woman can only have each birth experience once, so it is important that she makes it the best birth she can.

Being On Call

Being on call is a true privilege, and a role that obviously has to be taken very seriously. It is almost impossible not to put your life on hold, thinking that at any moment labour will start and you will have to drop whatever you are doing and run. In my experience, it is unusual for a woman to go into labour when she is not relaxed and comfortable. This means that most begin during the late evening or early hours of the morning, when they know their birth partners are close by and available.

With my clients, I like to discuss the following scenarios:

- If labour starts in the middle of the night, and she doesn't need you, then she should ideally not wake you, or you will both become exhausted having been up all night.
- If labour begins during the daytime and she is at home alone, then she may feel safer calling you immediately, giving you plenty of time to organise whatever you need to before joining her. In this instance, you can arrive before she requires support, but try to stay out of her way.
- If journey times, weather or traffic concerns are applicable, agree on a plan that will ease her mind about you making it to the birth on time. In my case, as I may have to drive up to an hour away to attend a birth, I like to make sure that my client knows she can contact me when she needs me, no matter what time of day or night. If, let's

say, that time was approaching rush hour, or there was a weather warning, I encourage her to call me out earlier, and I could perhaps sleep on her sofa or in a spare room. This kind of plan is particularly important for a second or subsequent baby, whose birth may happen faster than a first baby's.

On Call Dos and Don'ts

- **Do make sure she feels safe, warm and loved.** If you can help her create a relaxed and calm state of mind, you will be encouraging her to let go of fear, and her hormones will be at optimal levels.

- **Do remind her that the baby will come when it is ready.** It is thought that the baby will release a cocktail of hormones to signal the mother's body that it is ready to be born. The normal gestational period is between 37 and 42 weeks, but in my experience, most women are nearer 41 weeks when labour begins.

- **Don't ask her if she is feeling any signs of labour.** This puts her under pressure and reduces oxytocin.

- **Don't give her dates when she can or cannot have the baby, even jokingly.** Deadlines and dates when she is not allowed to go into labour will cause her stress and worry that you will not be available. If there is a date that is important to you, keep it to yourself and carry on as normal. In 99.9% of cases, the dates will not clash with the birth and all will be well.

- **Don't drink alcohol when you are on call.** I have met many women over the years who feel extremely anxious about going into labour when their birth partner has been drinking near the due date. From about 38 weeks onwards, it's best to avoid drinking alcohol altogether.

Discuss ways of communication, and agree on how you would like her to contact you. My rules are not to use 'What's App' during labour and never leave a voicemail—ever! If she needs an answer to a question quickly, she should call or send a text which will alert me immediately, and I will know that she needs me or needs an immediate response.

P. R. O. T. E. C. T. S.

This is an acronym I developed and have been teaching successfully for many years to hundreds of couples. Its intention is to help ensure that any birth partner can remember all the relevant parts of the role that could be considered their responsibility. This tool can be used during labour and also in the postnatal period.

**A birth partner PROTECTS the woman
no matter what type of birth she has.**

- **P**ositions: Make her comfortable, ideally with her pelvis upright and forward
- **R**efreshments: Encourage her to eat and drink regularly
- **O**xytocin: Keep room warm, dark, and private; make her feel safe and loved
- **T**iming: Time contractions only when necessary; be discreet
- **E**nvironment: Dim the lights, move the bed, play music, and use focal points
- **C**alm: Use breathing and relaxation skills, hypnobirthing techniques, and affirmations
- **T**ouch: Use massage, sacral pressure, anchors, and acupressure—if she consents
- **S**ilence: Be led by her, but try not to talk if possible

P: Positions

The position of a woman during labour is very important to the process of birth, so I have written a whole chapter on this subject (see Chapter 8). Please read it carefully, as it is the birth partner's job to make sure the woman they are supporting is comfortable during labour and birth, and in a position that will help her relax, encouraging the release of oxytocin. A good position will also create up to 30% more space which can facilitate the easiest possible route for the baby on its way through the pelvis.

R: Refreshments

You would not believe how many couples I have met who had a very difficult birth experience first time round, and when I un-picked what happened, I discovered that they didn't eat or drink during the entire labour and birth. They simply forgot, and had not made the connection to the fact that without food and water, the body simply can't function well, so the labour was long and tough. In this situation, contractions can slow down or stop completely, which will potentially lead the midwife or doctor to step in and administer synthetic drugs and/or IV fluids to bring the contractions back. Ideally, we want to ensure that this does not happen during the birth you attend. Whilst there is no doubt that the hardest job for a birth partner is to convince a labouring woman to eat when she simply doesn't fancy anything, you do have to try. Offer her small bite-sized pieces of food that are easy to eat, nutritious and something she loves, after a contraction has finished and when she is reasonably alert. If you notice her resting with her eyes closed, leave her alone and wait until the end of the next one. Any rest she can get between contractions conserves her energy.

Early Labour (0–4 cm)

In the early stages of labour, I recommend that she continues to eat and drink as normal. Most women begin labour at night and if she has had a good dinner the night before, then she should be ok to get up in the morning as usual and eat a good breakfast long before labour becomes established.

Established Labour (4–10 cm)

As labour progresses, offer small portions of something that will give her energy. Try not to ask her too often, but at least once an hour give her a small snack in between each contraction, perhaps a spoonful of yogurt or a small bite of banana.

Snack Ideas for your Birth Bag

Most people think that granola bars are the perfect snack to pack in a birth bag, when in reality they can be dry and chewy and therefore tricky to eat when there is limited time between contractions. So, prepare well in advance for the kinds of things that you know she likes. See the list below for some suggestions. I recommend that you discuss refreshments thoroughly with her in the antenatal period and ensure she understands that on the day, even if she tells you that she is not hungry, that she has to help you by eating something little and often.

- **Honey sticks.** These are small portions of honey packed into a straw which make for very easy consumption. You may need to take a pair of scissors to open these depending on the brand. They are an excellent way to get some natural sugar into a labouring woman. You can always just pack a pot of honey and a spoon.
- **Jelly pots.** Not necessarily the healthiest option, but useful as they last a long time and do not need to be kept in the fridge. Make sure you get the full sugar version.
- **Yogurt.** These are cold and refreshing, and if you don't have any, ask your midwife if she has one you can have.
- **Bananas.** Brilliant for a quick fix that will help to boost energy with no preparation necessary.

- **Chocolate.** This dissolves in the mouth so takes little effort to consume.
- **Runner's gel/isotonic gel.** These small flavoured sachets can be useful to squeeze into her mouth for an instant energy boost. They are very concentrated, so small, regular amounts are all that is required.
- **Dried fruit.** Give in small portions. Pack a knife or a pair of scissors to cut pieces up.
- **Ask your midwife** if there is any fresh food she can offer. I find that fresh fruit and yogurt are readily available in most hospitals and midwife-led units.
- **Granola bars.** I would suggest you have one or two in the bag as a back up, but don't rely on them completely as you may find she just cannot face the effort it takes to chew and swallow them.

Consider making food and freezing it so that you know it will stay cold and fresh for you both to snack on. Top recommendations, which can be packed in a very small coolbag (don't forget to take them with you when you go!):

- **Small smoothie shots.** Prepare small portions of fruit smoothies that are filled with berries, banana and yogurt and put them into little pots or an ice cube tray. They will defrost quicker, and you will only need to give her a small amount each time.
- **Frozen berries.** Blueberries are good (you can buy them pre-frozen if you prefer). They melt in the mouth when frozen, are cold and delicious to suck on when she is feeling hot, and provide an excellent energy boost.
- **Frozen sweets** such as Haribos or other jelly sweets. Chopped up pieces of chocolate bars are popular too.
- **Ice lollies.** These are the perfect way to cool her down and give her something sweet. A Solero is a particular favourite of my clients.

- **Frozen sandwiches.** If you like sandwiches, you can make them and freeze them in advance so that throughout labour you can help yourself to them without having to leave the room.

Consider avoiding food for yourself that has strong odours. Most women find that their sensitivity to smell is heightened during labour, so cheese and onion crisps are a big no! Choose your food wisely, and pack a toothbrush and toothpaste or some breath fresheners just in case.

What to Drink

It is very important that you both keep hydrated. When a woman is in labour, she is burning off a lot of fluids, so she needs to drink consistently. I advise you to buy a pack of bendy straws so that you can place the straw to her lips and she doesn't need to hold the drink herself. You will need two or three depending on how many different drinks she has throughout the birth.

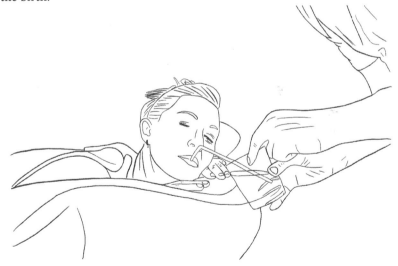

- Water is essential, and should be offered after every two or three contractions.
- Isotonic drinks can be refreshing.

- Coconut water gives energy and is very useful to pack in a birth bag.
- Squash. Remember to get the one that isn't sugar free!
- Try to avoid giving fizzy drinks if possible.

IMPORTANT TO KNOW *If gas and air is used during labour (see Chapter 12), it will really dry out her mouth, so she should be offered a drink at the end of every contraction.*

Burping and Vomiting

During labour, it is not uncommon for a woman to feel very 'gassy' and burp a lot. Some women will feel nauseous and others will actually vomit. Typically, this may only be once or twice, and whilst it can happen at any point, it is more likely to be towards the end of labour nearer transition. Sniffing lemon or lemon oil may help her to feel better. Rarely, I have supported women who have vomited throughout the entire labour, and these are the hardest of all to convince that they still need to eat and drink, as doing so makes them feel worse. In this instance, I recommend ice chips. You can fill a small food thermos, which should stay frozen for about 24 hours if not opened. Some women like soft sweets to suck on such as haribo, or chocolate drops, which can also be frozen in advance of labour and melt on the roof of the mouth.

Going to the Toilet

A full bladder can affect the baby moving downwards, so once labour becomes established, be sure to suggest she go to the toilet at least every hour or two. As the baby moves down, and a woman begins to push, the bowel can be squashed near the entrance of the rectum. A woman may pass poo at this stage if she hasn't already emptied her bowels before or during the labour. Don't be surprised; this is perfectly normal and the midwife will cover it or remove it as a matter of routine. Some women never even know about it, so it is your job to say nothing—unless she asks.

O: Oxytocin

In labouring women, oxytocin is necessary to produce contractions and dilate the cervix. Levels increase when a woman feels safe, warm and loved. A dark environment works best for privacy, which is why many women will begin labour in the middle of the night. The birth partner is responsible for protecting oxytocin so that labour can progress (see Chapter 4), as it is very easily knocked out by the hormone adrenaline. You need to identify if there are specific ways that you can help the woman you are supporting to relax. Talking to her about what she thinks might increase adrenaline— thoughts, fears, doubts—and having an action plan of ways to help her to let go of negative thoughts and tension will help keep her oxytocin levels high. By thoroughly understanding the role of both of these hormones, and how each one affects the labour, a woman is much more likely to have a quicker and more straightforward birth experience.

T: Timing

Labouring women should not focus on the time. The birth partner doesn't need to either, but if anyone is going to do it, it must be you. There is a terrible tendency to analyse the labour far too much when you are timing contractions. Questions such as 'Was that one longer or shorter than the last one?', 'Do you think they are getting closer together?' or 'Are they getting stronger?' mean that you are both on high alert all the time. When it comes to timing contractions, my top tip is don't. Only begin timing when she starts telling you that she is wondering if you should call the midwife. Only then is it a good idea to sit quietly for about 10 minutes, making a note of what she is experiencing in order to get a picture of what is going on. Even just seeing you looking at your watch can be off-putting for her.

The birth partner should observe the labouring woman and look for the following three things.

1. Length

2. Strength

3. Distance between

Length. Most contractions at the start of labour last 20–30 seconds. They will lengthen as the labour progresses. Short contractions are over pretty quickly—the woman is back to normal immediately afterward, and I would describe her as 'back in the room'. As the labour begins to ramp up, you will easily begin to sense that her contractions are getting longer without having to time them. As the sensations build, she will begin to focus on her breathing more intently, and will need some recovery time. Keep her calm and remind her to breathe if you notice she is forgetting.

Strength. It is very hard to tell what is happening for a woman regarding strength if she is not relaxed and calm. If she is caught up in the fear-tension-pain cycle (see Chapter 11), she might struggle to cope with the sensations. So, from the outset, a woman should be encouraged to get comfortable and to breathe. Her ability to cope well in the early stages will set the scene for the labour as it progresses. It is vital that she is able to rest between the surges to conserve energy when possible, and it will then become more noticeable when her labour is ramping up. She will express to you that the contractions feel stronger and you will see her behaviour change when they do. Try not to engage with her at all if you can, other than to offer her something to eat or drink. Again, the best way to describe what you are looking for is to ask yourself how quickly she is 'back in the room'. When each surge ends, notice what she's doing.

- In early labour, she will be capable of going straight back to whatever she was doing before the contraction started.
- In established labour, she will take a while to recover and will be unable to talk much in between.
- In the later stages, she will most likely be able to hear everything going on around her, but will be in her own little world. Leave her

there, as this is a very important time, and if you keep bringing her back into the room, the labour will be long and exhausting.

Distance between. This is the one that most people focus on. They are trained by books and antenatal courses to look out for contractions that come around three or four every 10 minutes, lasting at least a minute. Whilst this is a good guide, it is not a one-size-fits-all recommendation, and some women will never fall into that ratio. I once had a client whose contractions came every six minutes and lasted 45 seconds and she gave birth easily. So my top tip is to look out for regularity. Over time, her sensations will start to form a noticeable pattern that you could set your watch by. If she is having short ones, then long ones, then back to short with gaps that are randomly spaced, then she is not quite there yet. You want the pattern to be consistent, with approximately the same distance between. She needs to be totally focused on the surges and take time to recover afterwards.

A Rough Guide to Timings

Your midwife will be wanting you to call them out for a home birth, or leave home and head to the hospital, around the time that the contractions are as follows (remember that this is a rough guide!).

1. Length: Each contraction lasts about one minute long.

2. Strength: She is having to completely focus on her breath.

3. Distance between: They are approximately two to three mins apart, and she is having at least three contractions in every 10 minutes.

E: Environment

Hopefully labour will begin at the woman's home, so she is in complete control of her environment during the earlier stages of labour. If she is remaining at home for her birth, then nothing needs to change. If she is using a birth pool, then you can begin to fill it in preparation for her to want to use it. If this is a first baby, you can wait until her contractions are regular and forming a pattern, so start as soon as you are confident that labour is establishing. If it is a second or subsequent baby, begin filling the pool as soon as you are aware that she is in labour, because it can take an hour or more in some cases, and it would be a shame if the baby came before the pool was ready. If she is giving birth in an MLU or hospital, and she wants to use water, be sure to mention it on the phone when you call. I often ask the midwife to start filling the pool in preparation for our arrival, which many are happy to do.

In the event that you are in a regular hospital room with a bed in the middle, then you will want to take control of the environment as soon as possible after arriving. Ideally you can try and re-create what you were doing at home.

This may include:

- Getting her into a good position.
- Getting her drinks and snacks ready.
- Switching off the lights.
- Putting on some music.
- Moving the room around to ensure that it works for you rather than the other way around.

Look for the controls on the side panel of the bed, and use the buttons to raise or lower the bed into the right position for her. I recommend that you sit her on an exercise ball and raise the bed up to a higher level so that she can lean over the bed and rest forward.

IMPORTANT TO KNOW *Most hospitals and MLUs have exercise balls, and you can check this if you go on a hospital visit or give them a call to ask what they have available for use. I recommend you also consider taking your own, or if possible take a pump so that if theirs are too small or soft, you can blow them up a bit more.*

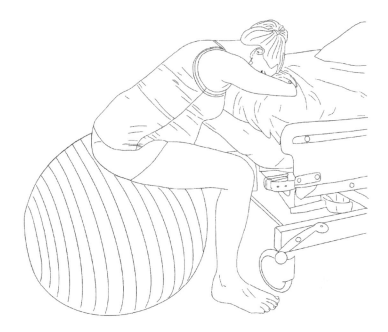

If labour begins in hospital after an induction, then all the above still applies. From the outset, take control of the room or curtained bay in the ward by organising what you need to create a lovely calm environment for her and get her comfortable. My advice is to avoid long walks as these can be very tiring. Lots of rest will help raise her oxytocin levels, which is what you need to get contractions going. Obviously there is no harm in going out for some fresh air and a short walk, but you do not want to exhaust her too early in the process.

C: Calm

Keeping yourself calm. Many women will describe that in the postnatal period that they spent the entire labour worrying about their birth partner. They describe being unable to relax because they could tell the person beside them wasn't coping. Whether you are a spouse, parent, sibling or friend, if you are going to attend a birth with any labouring woman, you should look at ways you can remain calm during the birth, so that you can protect her oxytocin. This book speaks a lot about ways to ensure that the labouring woman is well informed and well supported, but what if *you* have questions, worries or concerns about what is happening in any given moment, and *you* have fears and doubts about whether she is coping, or if she and the baby are ok? First, if you think that you are going to struggle, you should definitely consider asking a doula or another experienced person who is confident and understands the process of birth to join your team. They will be able to give you both lots of reassurance on the day. Second, you can practice relaxation techniques yourself in advance of the birth to help you know how to switch off and let go of trying to 'fix' birth, which is one of the most common issues for anyone to feel when they are beside a labouring woman. And last, if you are ever worried or have questions about something that is happening within the labour, don't ignore that feeling. Go and find a midwife or a doctor who will give you some answers quickly, or in the case of being at home in early labour, phone the labour ward number or midwifery team. The sooner that you can let go of your own worries and stress, the sooner you will be able to offer appropriate support to her.

Keeping her calm. It is an important part of a birth partner's role to be able to keep a labouring woman calm when she is beginning to wobble. The sensations that she is feeling will become longer and stronger. This can cause her to feel like she is losing control as the labour ramps up. It is important to remind her that she is doing great, that you are beside her and can help her to get through each surge. If the average length of a contraction is approximately one minute long during the active phase, then each time she begins to feel a sensation start, you can help her slow her breathing down. Focusing on each breath, rather than the actual contraction, works like magic and will help her to regain a sense of calm.

IMPORTANT TO KNOW *If she is already breathing well, please don't give her tips on how to breathe calmly. Trust me, this is very annoying and will reduce her oxytocin. The plan is that you only step up if she is struggling—I call this 'being, not doing'.*

When each contraction has finished, encourage her to rest forward, relax all the muscles in her body and breathe in and out through her nose. I find essential oils like lavender can work well to help keep her calm. Put some onto a tissue that can be removed from the room if she doesn't like it. Some smells can be repugnant to women in labour, even when they have loved them previously. The tissue can be removed from the room immediately if she hates it. Homeopathic remedies, such as pulsatilla or aconite, can be effective too in handling the emotional side of labour. Ensure you keep them separate from any essential oils, so as not to harm their potency, as strong scents can cancel out the effects. Playing soft, relaxing music can make a huge difference at this time to keep a woman calm. I find that most women want tracks without words; however, some want to have upbeat, uplifting tunes that they can sing to. If using specific hypnosis tracks, she might prefer to use headphones and truly get into the zone.

T: Touch

I find that during an antenatal discussion, when I talk about touch, most women are delighted to hear that they might experience a lovely massage, or be held and stroked in labour. If she agrees, practice a few moves together in the antenatal period. This will enable you both to become familiar with what she likes, and where on her body she is happy to be touched. Sometimes, a woman's feelings change, and those who were most looking forward to that massage actually hate you touching them once labour is underway, as their body is too sensitive. As the baby moves down and through her pelvis, the sensations can become overwhelming, and what was once the right pressure in the right place will become the wrong pressure in the wrong place. Discuss the idea of a signal that she can use to make you "STOP" whenever she needs you too; I always suggest she raises a hand. Sometimes I will be told by a woman from the outset that she would not like to be touched, and it is important to remember this on the day and respect her physical boundaries. Occasionally, a woman who would normally hate to be touched in any way will actually need lots of hugs and love, so be prepared to have an open mind, and encourage her to have a flexible mindset too. Make sure that if she changes her mind, she knows that she can communicate that clearly to you, so you know exactly what she requires on the day of birth.

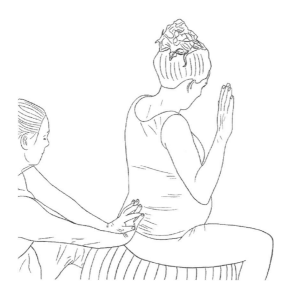

Massage Techniques

Massage techniques release endorphins, and here are some popular strokes to use between contractions to help her to relax:

* Light touch massage. Stroke your partner softly using your fingertips. You can lightly stroke her neck, across her shoulders and down her back using one hand or both to create a lovely tingling feeling.

- Nerve strokes. Using a little more pressure, stroke down each side of the back alternating hands, always keeping one hand on her back at all times. This is lovely to do between contractions.
- Shaking the apples. Using one clenched fist on each bum cheek, make circles with your fists to shake or jiggle the buttocks. This can loosen any tension and relax the muscles in and around the woman's hips, and pelvis.

The following techniques are particularly useful to use during a contraction, providing an action that can help alleviate the sensations or open the pelvis:

- Figure of 8. Draw a side-lying figure of 8 using one or two hands around the lower part of her back to provide a pleasant pressure over the sacrum. Ask her for feedback in case she would like you to use more pressure.
- Sacral pressure. Using two hands, press all your weight into her lower back to relieve pressure in the sacrum. With sacral pressure, she might like you to put pressure on her sacrum at the start of each sensation, but at the peak, it might feel too intense. A rhythm may begin to develop that ensures you start the pressure, and then when she signals you to stop, you do so quickly and easily. As the sensation begins to diminish, she may signal for you to start again until the contraction is over. A clear method of communicating can really help to ensure that you get into a pattern that is easy for you both to understand.
- Double hip squeeze. During a contraction, point your fingertips inwards and lean in with your body weight to squeeze her hips together (see Figure 9.1, on the next page). This can help to splay open the pelvis at the outlet to create more room for the baby.

IMPORTANT TO KNOW   *If a woman is using a TENS machine for pain relief, it is much harder to use touch techniques for support. In this scenario, I recommend you stick to upper back strokes, and stroke down the neck, shoulders and arms.*

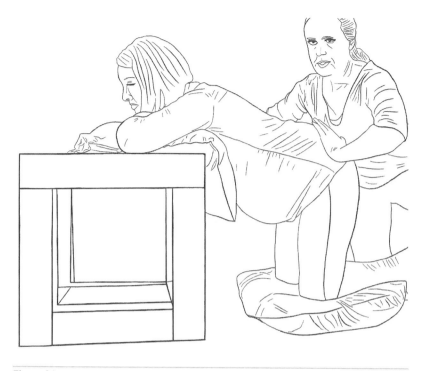

Figure 9.1

S: Silence

As the birth partner, it is important for you to remember that too much talking in a birth room can reduce the production of oxytocin. Often women don't realise the impact it can make. However, this is not true for all women, so I therefore recommend that you follow her lead. Only talk if she is talking to you—otherwise you stay quiet. If you think she is becoming distracted by too much talking, then you will need to do what I call 'shut the room down' and make a point of staying quiet. Perhaps encourage her to listen to relaxing music, or you could break a conversation by telling her you have to leave the room for a minute or two and then when you come back in, you remain quiet. This is also especially important for those who are attending the birth with you (midwives/care assistant/doctors). It is not always easy for your care providers to stay quiet, but it is your job, as the birth partner, to ask them to if it is distracting her.

IMPORTANT TO KNOW *If you are already aware that she may be distracted by noise, then encourage the use of headphones. She can also state at the very top of her birth plan that she is hypnobirthing, which will help her care providers to recognise that she doesn't want anyone to talk around her.*

Lower the Tone

If the woman you are supporting would like everyone around her to be quiet, then make sure to lead by example. When you arrive at the hospital, or when the midwife arrives at a home birth, speak quietly from the outset. This will set the tone for the type of behaviour that you are looking for, and it is important to stick with that throughout. If a doctor or midwife enters the room and begins a conversation whilst a contraction is happening, always wait until the contraction has gone before you reply. Then always reply in a whisper. Don't be tempted to break this rule, as it can add many hours to the birth. Women need high levels of oxytocin for progress to be made in labour, and if you are having a conversation in the background while she is labouring, it will be distracting and can easily cause adrenaline levels to rise.

IMPORTANT TO KNOW *It is not uncommon for a doctor or midwife to actually try and have a conversation with a woman in the middle of a contraction. In this instance, she should know that she can raise her hand and not attempt to answer them until she has recovered.*

Being not Doing

I want to end this chapter by sharing with you that the best possible birth companion is someone who can truly understand the concept of being present with a woman in labour, by having the ability to sit on their hands and not try to 'fix' the birth for her. Throughout the chapters in this book, my intention is to help you learn that 'less is more' and 'if it ain't broke, don't fix it'.

The PROTECTS tool is simple and easy to use, and a shortened version is available as a free download with this book. Be sure to print it out and keep it handy to refer to on the day. This will help you remember that if she is calm and comfortable, getting regular snacks and drinks, and using the toilet every hour or two, then you can sit beside her and do very little if all is going smoothly: what doulas call 'being, not doing'.

If at any point during the labour things begin to change, then you will know how and when to step up and provide her with more emotional and/ or physical support. I call this 'reading the room'.

A good birth partner will benefit by staying quiet, keeping calm, and resting when she is resting.

IMPORTANT TO KNOW *I recommend that you avoid using your mobile phone during the labour. Where possible, try to avoid any communication with friends and family. This can really put the labouring woman under pressure to perform, and she will be aware that your focus is elsewhere, which can be very distracting.*

* *

CLAIRE'S STORY Claire's mum wanted to be at her birth. She knew deep down that her mum would stress her out, so she had kindly explained that she wouldn't be invited. Her mum was disappointed, but asked if Claire would let her know the minute labour started, so she could feel involved from a distance. As promised, Claire messaged her mum when her waters broke at 4.30 AM and kept in touch with her throughout the day. Her contractions were slow and didn't really get going until it was dark outside later that night. By the time Claire was ready to go to the hospital, it was 6 AM the following morning. She was exhausted and had had little sleep for two nights. Claire knew her mum was worried, and it had played on her mind. As labour progressed into day two, her partner was able to update her mum, but had to leave the room to get a signal which was annoying and distracting. All that day, her mum had been messaging asking for updates,

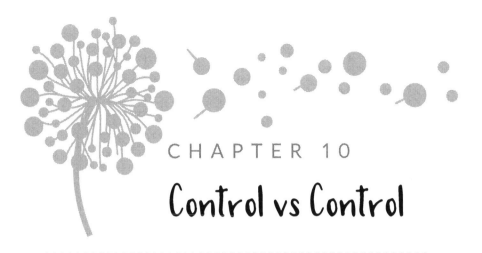

CHAPTER 10

Control vs Control

Your body can withstand almost anything. It's your mind you have to convince.

–Ina May Gaskin

I'm sure it's no surprise to hear that many modern women like to be in control of their lives. Certainly a significant number of the pregnant women I meet in my classes or as doula clients admit to being careful planners who thrive on organisation and structure. When it comes to having a baby, however, the fact that many women are led by their left brain (the part of the brain that manages logic) means that they might struggle to let go of control on the day of their birth. This can be tricky because, as mammals, we are not designed to overthink or overanalyse our bodies' ability to give birth. You wouldn't find a female gorilla worrying about how on earth she is going to cope in labour, or see a cat getting worked up about what position she needs to adopt for her kittens to be born safely. So this chapter should help you, as the birth partner, to understand when control in a birth room is necessary and, more importantly, when it is not.

There are some obvious things that she can be in control of that affect the birth positively, such as choosing the right people to attend and support her, being prepared and knowledgeable about the process of giving birth, learning to breathe and relax anytime she chooses to, and having the confidence to know that nothing can be done to her during the birth unless it is approved by her first. However, what many women in labour don't realise is that they can also try to control the process in a negative way. This happens when they constantly overanalyse what is happening to them during the birth itself, which of course has a direct impact on the production of birth hormones if adrenaline is triggered too early. It is, therefore, very important that you are able to understand and recognise if the woman you are supporting is trying to control her birth. By learning the difference between positive and negative control, you will know that if she is, you can step in and act. This is the time when too much excitement and overstimulation can literally knock off progress, leading to a longer and more difficult labour overall.

Negative Control

When a woman 'overthinks' during her labour, she will produce adrenaline. She is controlling her thoughts constantly and is completely unable to switch off and listen to her body. Because of the effect this has on oxytocin production, she may struggle to progress smoothly and easily in labour, and it can become difficult and more painful—she is simply too 'present in the room'. It is hard as a birth partner to prevent this, but you do have to try.

Examples of a woman who is controlling her birth negatively can include: a woman who tells everyone she is in labour and is on Facebook groups asking questions; a woman who is unable to switch off her mobile phone; a woman who wants to time her contractions and then analyses; a woman who is distracted by the simplest things (sounds in the background, certain words spoken, an inability to get comfortable). She may also have anxiety due to a previous negative birth experience or trauma.

If you already know that it might be a problem for the woman you are supporting to let go of controlling everything around her during labour, and she is always overthinking, I would recommend you both attend some hypnobirthing classes together (see Chapter 11). It is one of the easiest ways to prepare a woman mentally for the upcoming birth, helping her and you as her birth partner to understand the importance of relaxation, and how the body does not respond well when a labouring woman is too 'in her own head'. She will learn vital tools to enable her to switch off the thinking part of her brain, and you will learn skills to support her in doing this.

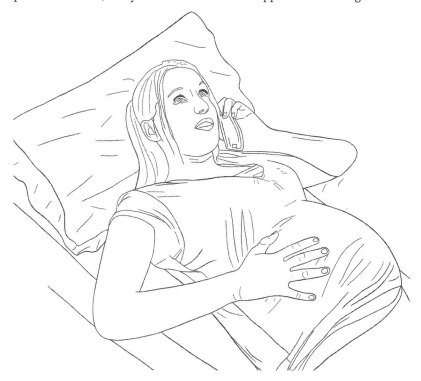

Follow Her Lead

If, during the labour, she wants to engage and have a conversation with you, then of course it is ok to speak to her. Ideally, though, you should just follow her lead and answer any questions she asks you in a calm and casual manner, whilst staying quiet the rest of the time. Make sure that you don't engage in heavy discussions and try not to ask her any questions. This is especially important when offering food or drink. She will decline the offer if she doesn't want the refreshments, but at least you are not asking her questions all the time that require a response.

It is better to say:

- 'Here is your drink', rather than 'can I get you a drink?'
- 'Have a bite of this', rather than 'would you like a snack?'
- 'Your cold flannel is here when you need it', rather than 'can I get you a cold flannel?'

If she asks you questions about her progress, your answers should be short and reassuring. For example:

- Question: Do you think that the contractions are getting longer?
- Answer: They seem perfect to me.
- Question: Have you fed the dog?
- Answer: No need to worry, I have everything sorted.
- Question: I am worried that the contractions are not getting closer together.
- Answer: That's ok—as long as you are resting in between, that's all that matters.
- Question: Can you call the hospital and ask them when they think we should go?
- Answer: If you are ok, and you are feeling the baby move regularly, then I think we should try to stay at home for as long as we can. (You will know it's time to go to the hospital, because she won't even want to ask you questions—she will be telling you she needs to go!)

. . . .

ANJA'S STORY I went to Anja's home during the birth of her second baby. When I arrived at 3 AM, Anja and her husband were both in their brightly lit kitchen chatting whilst he emptied the dishwasher. Apparently labour had slowed a little since she had called me to come over, and so they were just hanging out. I took a little bit of time to notice what was going on, and it was obvious that they were in entertainment mode and were asking me: Can I get you a drink? Do you want something to eat? What do you think we should do next? After about 15 minutes of catching-up time, I gradually began to reduce the level of my voice, and then suggested that it would be nice to go and get comfortable. I took her to the lounge, switched out the lights and put on some relaxation music and stopped all conversation. Within 10 minutes, her contractions were back and within the hour, she was in full blown labour. Her husband had inadvertently slowed her labour down by throwing a party in the middle of the kitchen at 3 AM. If she had remained upstairs in their dark quiet bedroom after she called me, and he had gone downstairs alone, her contractions might not have slowed. Be mindful of your own role in this birth scenario and protect the oxytocin at all times.

• •

Examples of Negative Control

- Overthinking
- Timing contractions
- Analysing what is happening to her contractions during her labour (too short, too weak, too irregular)
- Consistently engaging with those around her
- Using her mobile phone
- Asking lots of questions
- Being unable to relax or get comfortable

Positive Control

Making a list of birth preferences is a constructive way for a pregnant woman to remain in positive control (see Chapter 13). If she can identify and document the type of birth she is interested in achieving, then she can share those with you and her care providers. This will enable her to let go of that particular element of control, knowing that all her wishes are there for you to refer to if necessary. Focusing on breathing and relaxation during labour will help to keep her mind off the actual sensations she is experiencing. It's so important for her to try to stay out of her 'thinking brain'. If she forgets to breathe and starts to lose focus, you will notice and be right there to remind her. It is also important for her to know that she can use her voice in labour if she needs to. I always remind women of this in pregnancy, as many think they won't be able to talk at all. Women can get their needs across quickly and efficiently by saying simple instructions like 'water', 'snack', 'stop talking', or 'not right now'. If she can't or doesn't want to vocalise, then tell her to raise a hand if there is something she wants you to stop doing immediately, such as talking or touching her. If a decision does need to be made during the labour that is not included on her list of preferences, then you can of course involve her in a brief discussion. Chances are, if things get to that stage, she will be instinctively aware that something is not right. Chapter 15, which covers 'Plan B', will help you understand what to do in this scenario.

Examples of Positive Control
- Making a list of birth preferences ahead of time
- Using breathing and relaxation techniques
- Practicing hypnobirthing
- Getting into comfortable positions
- Making decisions around her preferences and asserting them
- Finding her voice if required, or raising a hand to ask others around her to be quiet

The Need for Certainty

Whilst there is absolutely nothing wrong with a woman planning and preparing for her baby's arrival, it's important to know that, deep down, what she might be seeking is certainty—that the labour will be short or long, easy or hard, simple or complicated. Any birthing woman and her partner should understand that, when it comes to giving birth, there are no guarantees. If during the labour she asks you questions to which she wants a definitive answer, such as 'how much longer will this take', you should never give her a response that indicates certainty. I see many birth partners make the mistake of saying 'this baby will be here by midnight, I promise' and then the woman is devastated when midnight comes and goes and there is no sign of the baby. In my experience, women who struggle with lack of certainty the most are more likely to accept an induction more readily, or will choose to have a planned c-section because it eliminates uncertainty, especially around when the baby will be born. If this is true for the woman you are supporting, then that is absolutely fine; you will be able to move forward knowing that this is the case, and she will find it easier coping simply because she has a plan. Help her to get everything organised and make the planning as special as you can so that she feels nurtured and knows you are there for her.

Estimated Due Date

Estimated (adjective)

roughly calculated; approximate (of a value or number).

The date that a woman is given to estimate when her baby will be born is thought to be approximately 280 days, or 40 weeks starting from the first day of her last menstrual period. The midwife usually calculates the estimate due date (EDD) at the booking-in visit; however, it is not unusual for it to be changed by a sonographer at the 12-week 'dating' scan. Once given, a woman's due date becomes imprinted in her mind and, as her pregnancy develops, this date becomes a big focus for her. She may talk about whether she thinks the baby will be 'early' or 'late', putting great emphasis on that date, when in reality her baby could come anytime between 37 and 42 weeks. No matter how often women hear the words 'babies come when they are ready', most still secretly believe that their baby will be born early, so any day after their EDD can feel like a lifetime.

Looking at the statistics, I can tell you that:

- Around 11% of babies will be born before 37 weeks.
- Around 80% of babies will be born between 38-42 weeks.
- Around 5-10% of babies will be born after 42 weeks.
- Only 4-5% of babies will be born on their actual due date.

Normal gestational length also varies with race and ethnicity, with evidence suggesting that black and Asian women are more likely to give birth around 39 weeks, whereas with white women, the median was 40 weeks.

Babies Come When They Are Ready

If the woman you are supporting arrives at her EDD with no sign of labour, be guided by her. Tell her how beautiful she looks, raise her oxytocin with love and massage, go on short walks with her, and encourage her to meet up with her closest friends to pass the time. Reassure her that the baby will know when it is time to be born. You could also recommend that she connects with the baby either silently or vocally to strengthen the bond between them. It is hard to prepare women for any number of days past their EDD, and each day has the potential to feel long and exhausting for a woman who is in what I call the 'bring it on' phase of her pregnancy. She is ready and she wants her baby out, and the threat of induction is looming. She needs to maintain trust in her body above all else at this time, so keep reminding her how clever you think her body is.

> A woman does not have to give up control during labour; she just has to control the right elements.

The 'Bring It On' Phase

Most women eventually reach this phase at some point during the pregnancy. She feels as though she is bursting at the seams, and she wants her body back. She no longer dwells on how painful labour might be—she just wants to get the baby out and will literally do or try anything! As hard as those last weeks or days are for her, natural induction methods are still an intervention, and best described as 'ways to evict the baby before it is ready to be born'. In my experience literally nothing works if the baby is not ready, so if you can, remind her of how special these last days are so that she can practice relaxation, read, breathe deeply, eat nourishing food and rest as much as possible—the baby will be here before she knows it.

Natural Induction Methods

Despite that reminder, most women will still want to research and attempt things that encourage labour to begin. My advice is to try to find ways to encourage natural alignment in her body to give the baby the best chance to adopt a good position, as it is thought this can support the birth process. A rebozo (large shawl) can be used to help 'sift' the baby into a good position and can relax muscles, ligaments and tight fascia (connective tissue) in the mother. You can view examples of these sifting methods on Sophie Messager's website (**sophiemessager.com**) alongside other techniques on the Spinning Babies website (**spinningbabies.com**). A pregnancy-trained Bowen therapist, osteopath, or chiropractor can really make a big difference during the last weeks of pregnancy by aligning the mother's body, and most treatments are very relaxing. An acupuncturist, reflexologist or homeopath can also be useful in preparing a woman's body for giving birth, and have their own individual ways of stimulating labour depending on how pregnant the woman is at the time of the visit. Sex, nipple stimulation, and orgasm are thought to work if the baby is ready to be born, by triggering an abundance of hormones and helping blood flow to the genitals. Drinking raspberry leaf tea is thought to strengthen or ripen the uterus, and eating foods like spicy curry, dates and pineapple are all useful to open her bowels, which may encourage labour to start. Some women will swear that the methods they tried worked well if labour began soon afterwards, whereas others will be disappointed that nothing worked no matter how hard they tried.

QUICK RECAP

Here are the main things to remember when discussing control.

- **Positive and negative control.** Understand the difference between positive and negative control, knowing that she has the ability to remain in control of certain aspects of her birth experience.

- **Be honest.** Look closely at any areas that you think the woman you are supporting may struggle with. Sometimes a really honest discussion will need to take place.

- **Tell no one.** Talk about the use of social media or contacting friends or family members. It can be incredibly distracting for her (or you) to be on the phone.

- **Babies come when they are ready.** Remind her of this if she is struggling with the uncertainty of when the baby will be born and what the birth will eventually be like.

- **Praise and validate.** Remember to praise her and validate all the decisions she makes in any given moment. In some cases, she may want to or need to change her mind about her Plan A, so a flexible mindset is helpful.

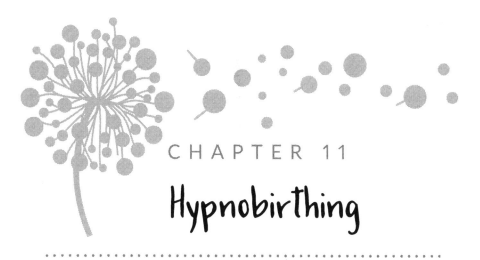

CHAPTER 11

Hypnobirthing

When you change the way you view birth, the way you birth will change.

–Marie Mongan

Hypnosis is a trance-like state that can be achieved when using deep breathing and relaxation. The name originates from the mid-19th century when Dr James Braid coined the term after the Greek God of sleep, Hypnos. Through the power of hypnosis, a willing participant's subconscious thoughts can be altered in a positive way. The subconscious mind, which is said to occupy around 90% of our brain capacity, includes our creative and spiritual sides, intuition, and long-term memory. Anything we have ever seen, experienced or heard about during our lifetimes is stored there. In a pregnant woman's subconscious, there may be negative stories about birth from well-meaning friends, along with passive visual images from the media of women lying on their backs with their legs in the air. These images can instill fear and doubt into the minds of modern-day pregnant women. Hypnobirthing—a term first credited in 1987 to Michelle Leclaire O'Neill, who published a book of the same name—is a tool that enables the woman to learn how to access her own subconscious mind so that she can reframe negative thoughts stored there. With the additional use of anchors and visualisation, she can use hypnobirthing as a safe and effective pain-management technique.

Power of the Mind

When in a hypnotic state, often compared to daydreaming, the woman is fully conscious but can tune out of the distractions around her. By learning about the power of her mind and how it connects to her body's functions in relation to the hormones she releases during labour, the woman and her birth partner can be empowered in their own roles and responsibilities in the process of giving birth.

The Stress Response

The effects of stress on the body are something that modern women (and men) are dealing with on a daily basis, even if they don't realise it. Stress can show up as anxiety, tension, difficulty sleeping, skin conditions, indigestion, constipation, painful periods, depression and much more, and is likely caused by the pressures we have in our busy lives in the modern world. The body's response to stress is physical, just like when our ancestors encountered a sabre-tooth tiger appearing at the door of their cave. We experience the fight-or-flight response, and blood is pumped away from the heart, and down to the limbs to enable our body to run from danger. If this happens during labour and birth because a woman is feeling stressed and fearful, there is reduced blood flow to her uterus because it is not deemed to be a necessary organ in that moment. Her production of oxytocin is wiped out by adrenaline, and dilation of the cervix is affected. If the woman has already perceived birth to be traumatic and painful, she will be proved right. If she is unable to relax, her levels of adrenaline will remain high, and she will stay in a permanent state of fight-or-flight mode. No oxytocin = no progress. This means that her birth is likely to be extremely challenging for her. The more fearful a woman is, the more tense she is, and therefore the more painful her birth will be—becoming a self fulfilling prophecy.

The Fear–Tension–Pain Cycle

When we feel fear in the body, it is held within our tissues—in every fibre of our being. Women fear the pain of labour because it is unknown. It can become massively built up in their minds, and many women will write themselves off from the outset. They say things like 'I will never cope with labour' and think their ability to cope has something to do with their pain threshold or stamina. Trust me, it doesn't! Dr Grantley Dick-Read, author of the book *Childbirth Without Fear*, found that women can get stuck in a cycle of fear, which leads to tension. This will inevitably cause them more pain. In 1916, he wanted to study women from poorer communities with little or no education, because they normally had simple, easy births, whereas the women from more affluent backgrounds cried out in agony. He determined the difference was all fear driven and developed his theory of the fear–tension–pain cycle. As fear creeps in, tension builds, and the pain cycle takes over (see Figure 11.1)

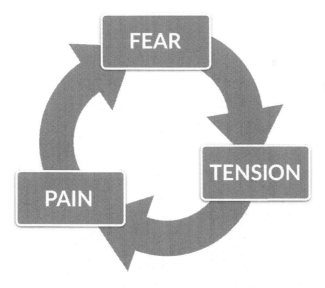

Figure 11.1 The right support can decrease fear, which decreases tension and therefore reduces pain.

The Basics of Hypnobirthing

If a woman can minimise her fears by using hypnobirthing methods in the antenatal period to change her mindset, she can have a completely different experience. This is achieved by training the brain to stay calm and relaxed. By accessing the subconscious mind through hypnosis, any woman can begin to reframe her thoughts. Changing those thoughts will help her to overcome her fears and find a way to feel confident. The results will be unique, depending on the course method, content chosen, and the level of time and effort she is able to commit whilst she practices these methods antenatally. Whether she invests in a few hypnosis tracks, an online programme, or a face-to-face course, it is important to use the techniques taught by the course provider regularly. As the birth partner, you can help by encouraging her to listen to the pre-recorded scripts, use visualisations, establish some anchors, and write out positive affirmations. All of these skills should soon start to feel familiar to you both if you are able to go through them together. On the day, she can then focus on a more beneficial cycle, like relax–calm–breathe (see Figure 11.2).

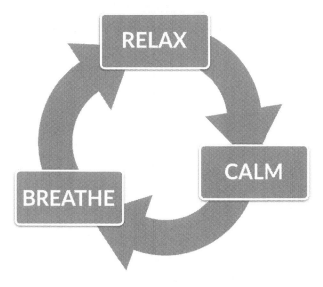

Figure 11.2 The right support increases the ability to relax, stay calm, and breathe.

Scripts

Most hypnobirthing courses will come with access to free scripts for you to read to her and/or pre-recorded tracks that she can listen to regularly. These will be aimed at easing her into a deep state of hypnosis and accessing her subconscious mind. With practice, she will then be able to achieve self-hypnosis. The content of the scripts are generally aimed at helping the pregnant woman retain a calm mindset, and to instill positive thoughts about her ability to give birth quickly and easily. Encourage her to listen often, and make sure to download these scripts on any devices that will be used at the birth so that they can be found and listened to easily on the day. I have included a free hypnobirthing track with this book (see the Resources section at the back of the book).

Visualisations

Many women love to use visualisations in labour to take themselves off somewhere else—a sandy beach, a mountain path, a favourite room. Others prefer to imagine the sensations they feel are coming and going like waves, flowing in and out like the tide. If they can actually see the pictures in their mind, then they are doing it right. Knowing and understanding her favourite visualisation will help you during labour if you notice that she needs support. By learning in advance what works for her, you can quickly take her back to a calm and relaxed state. For example, let's say she is beginning to forget to breathe deeply and starts telling you she is struggling. Get down to her level and speak quietly in the way that you practiced. It might sound like this: *It is a beautiful warm sunny day, and you are at the beach. As you walk along, you feel the soft golden sand under your feet. You smile and run off towards the sea, laughing as the waves lap at your ankles. You are so calm and you breathe deeply as you listen to the sounds of the waves* . . . . It also might help to have a photo she can gaze at as she visualises the scene.

Anchors

Anchors are simple ways to ensure that your partner remains in a hypnotic, relaxed state. By using touch, words or smells, you can send her deeper into relaxation. This can be particularly helpful if you notice that she is starting to come into a more awakened state and her thoughts, doubts and questions are returning. During pregnancy, you need to establish where she holds tension, what words support her ability to relax, and what smells or other sensations she likes.

I recommend the following common anchors:

- Stroking down the shoulders
- Phrases such as 'scan down your body and breathe', 'relax your shoulders', 'soften your jaw'
- Smells, perhaps of an essential oil like lavender or lemon placed on some tissue or cotton wool.
- Descriptions of a favourite view or holiday setting
- Feelings of warmth
- Music or nature sounds
- The taste of a certain food or drink she enjoys

Once you have identified what anchors she thinks will work well for her, practice them every now and again. This will help you to tune into them instinctively on the day.

Affirmations

Affirmations are positive statements that can remind a pregnant woman to trust her own body and instincts. They are hugely beneficial in changing negative thought patterns in the brain. As mammals, we have a tendency to lean towards negative thoughts. We need this tendency for survival and are naturally suspicious and on the lookout for danger. Because of this negative bias, our brains pay more attention to negative thoughts than positive ones. So, for affirmations to be effective, we need to hear and see them regularly to strengthen those positive pathways in the brain.

I recommend that the woman you are supporting thinks of at least 3 fears or worries. Talking it through with you, she can turn those negative thoughts into positive affirmations, such as, 'I put all fear aside as I prepare for the birth of my baby' or 'feeling calm and relaxed eliminates fear'. She should then write them down and put them in visible places—fridge door, mirrors, her car dashboard—where they can be seen and read by her sub-conscious mind every day. Here are a few more examples.

Negative	Positive
I am worried I won't be able to cope in labour.	I trust myself to breathe and relax during labour.
I am not very confident giving birth.	I am strong and confident and I trust my body.
I don't want to lose control.	I will keep control by staying calm and relaxed.
I am scared I will find it hard to give birth.	I let go of fear, which helps my body give birth easily.

Hypnobirthing Classes

There are lots of different ways to access hypnobirthing. The couples I typically support attend classes locally, either in small groups of between two and six couples or one-to-one private classes. Other options include buying a book, downloading an app, or signing up to a pre-recorded online course. These methods provide simple ways of learning the basics about hypnobirthing and how to use it. They should also come with free or additional downloads for hypnosis-style tracks that the woman can listen to in preparation for labour and birth.

Here is a list of what a hypnobirthing course should cover:

* How hormones affect a labouring woman
* How stress affects the body (fight or flight)
* The difference between the conscious and the subconscious mind
* How the body and mind work together
* Identification of her thoughts and beliefs
* How she can reframe her thoughts and beliefs
* An in-depth look at the role of the birth partner
* How to use intended hypnosis at home, along with audio tracks to practice regularly

A good quality course, be it virtual or in-person, should leave a pregnant woman feeling confident in her own body's ability to birth her baby, confident that she has all the tools she needs during the birth process, and confident that she is prepared for all eventualities in case she decides to switch to Plan B or if an unpredicted problem arises during the birth.

'Pain-Free' Language

Some courses may try to sell you the idea that hypnobirthing can lead to a 'pain-free' experience. Whilst I do know a few women (fewer than I can count on one hand) who would describe their birth in this way, the majority do not share this perception. In reality, her expectation should only be to learn the correct breathing and relaxation techniques during the pregnancy and practise them regularly. The more she accesses her subconscious mind and reframes her thoughts, the more likely she is to have a truly positive birth. By staying calm and relaxed, she can minimise fear and tension, which will then reduce—not necessarily eliminate—pain (see Figure 11.2). Another common element that is taught on a hypnobirthing course is to avoid the use of words like 'contraction' or 'pain'. There is solid logic behind this. Normally these words are replaced with other words that describe what is happening, like 'surge', 'sensation' or 'wave'. These are great alternatives, but in my experience, it is highly likely that whilst at the birth, you are both going to hear all kinds of words used by your care providers, including 'pain' and 'contraction'. So I recommend encouraging the woman you are supporting not to be too precious about the words she hears, or she may be brought out of hypnosis during labour when she hears a word she has been avoiding. Lastly, a typical problem I hear about regularly is that during a hypnobirthing course, the teacher may confuse a woman by leading her to believe she doesn't have to push the baby out, and that her body will do it all by itself. This can often be misinterpreted as: 'Don't Push!' Please read Chapter 6 regarding the second stage of labour carefully. No woman should ever ignore her body's own natural urge to push, especially if this is her first baby. Support her in listening to and following her body's sensations. This means: no resisting, no holding back, no special breathing techniques—simply going with her own body's signs and signals that take over when the time is right. If the woman feels an overwhelming urge to push, then she should definitely be following this instinct.

> Pain during childbirth is purposeful and productive—not a sign that something is wrong

Here are some words from clients who have recently attended a hypnobirthing course.

Martin: We did a hypnobirthing course and met three other lovely couples. It was fascinating to learn about the reasons why my wife, Fiona, had so many inner doubts and fears. I enjoyed all aspects of the course, and as well as a tonne of information, there were practical elements too. We went into our birth with an open mind, and on the day, Fiona was able to play the birth tracks continuously using her headphones. I only spoke to her once or twice during labour, as she was definitely in 'the zone'. I could tell when things were progressing by the sounds she made, and she told me it gave her confidence knowing that I was right beside her.

Sue: My daughter asked me to be her hypnobirthing partner on the day she told me she was pregnant. I was thrilled to have a role and took it very seriously, doing lots of research. I found the information shared during the online course fascinating. We watched each video together and I loved practicing the scripts with her and seeing her relax after a long day at work. She became very skilled at letting go and it made a huge difference during the labour. I wish I had done something like this when I was having my children.

Kirsty: I found out about hypnobirthing during my pregnancy yoga class. I wanted to try it because I felt I had a low pain threshold and it sounded ideal. On the day of my birth, things didn't go as planned, but I was still able to use the techniques throughout the labour and my eventual c-section. I was amazed at how useful the techniques have been since then, too. I use them almost daily to help me remain calm and focused, particularly when I am tired. I know that the skills are deep down in my subconscious and I can easily tune into a relaxed state anytime I choose.

The secret to hypnobirthing is that it actually gives control back to the labouring woman, who probably hadn't realised she had it all along. Remember the saying from Glinda the good witch in the film "The Wizard of Oz"? 'You've always had the power, my dear—you just had to learn it for yourself.'

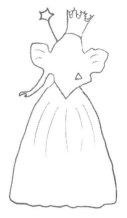

QUICK RECAP

Here are the main things to remember when discussing hypnobirthing.

- **Find a good course.** If hypnobirthing is something she is keen to use, find a good quality course that will help you both to learn how to use hypnosis.

- **Fear–tension–pain cycle.** Understand the concept of the fear-tension-pain cycle, so that she can release any fears she may be holding on to.

- **Breathe–calm–relax.** Learn the effects of the breathe-calm-relax alternative that supports the woman once negative beliefs are starting to diminish.

- **Affirmations.** Encourage her to write out three fears that she may have, and then brainstorm how she can turn them into positive affirmations.

- **Anchors.** Decide between you what anchors would work for her, such as touch, smell, sound, or sight. Learn these anchors to help you support her relaxation on the day of birth.

- **Practice.** Practice, practice, practice! Hypnobirthing scripts and hypnosis tracks are valuable as the pregnancy progresses. Try to use these tools daily from 36 weeks onwards.

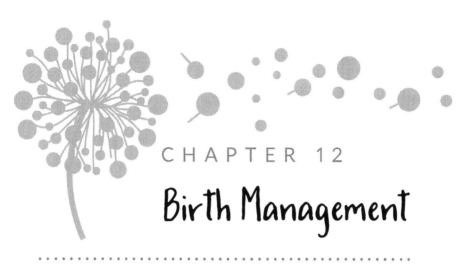

CHAPTER 12

Birth Management

Promise me you'll always remember you're braver than you believe, stronger than you seem, and smarter than you think.

—A. A. Milne

O btaining a woman's views on how she would like to manage her birth, including any pain relief methods she might be interested in using, is a top priority for any birth partner. During the birth planning sessions you schedule, you will have the opportunity to discuss her preferences about birth management in detail making sure you both know exactly what options are available to her. In this chapter, I will cover a variety of techniques and all methods of pain relief that are accessible to a woman depending on the location of her birth. It is important to discuss with her how she feels about each pain relief method available and then talk about whether it is a No, a Yes or a Maybe. In the next chapter, I will also share examples of how you can document these in a birth plan. This means that no birth partner need ever offer a labouring woman pain relief, and run the risk of undermining her confidence, because she will know what is available and request whatever she needs, whenever she is ready. The only time this may differ is when she specifically asks you to make suggestions, or she tells you she needs to be reminded of what is available for her.

Breathing

Breathing is the most powerful pain relief option there is in the early stages of labour, and it is helpful for a woman to concentrate on her breath during that time, regardless of whether she goes on to use other methods of pain relief or not. A woman who can distract herself from the sensations she is feeling and use her breath as a focus will find it easier to manage as labour progresses, and this will help her endorphin and oxytocin levels to rise. In particular, she will benefit from using her outbreath to really relax and let go, as it is very hard to tense up on a long exhalation. As labour continues, the woman may have moments where she feels overwhelmed and forgets to breathe altogether. If she is not supported during this time, she can begin to feel like she is completely losing control, and may even begin to scream out. Ideally we want to help her before this happens, so as her birth partner, your job is to remind her, or possibly even breathe with her in these moments. It can help to ask her in advance what she would prefer you to do.

Signs that she is holding tension and beginning to struggle might be her shoulders rising, or her vocalisations becoming more high pitched. If you see her losing control of her breath, quietly and simply stand close to her and say something like:

- 'Use your breath.'
- 'Take a nice deep breath in, and let this one go.'
- 'Would it help if I breathe with you?'

Focused Breathing Techniques for Early Labour

In early labour, breathing in a focused way is easy for the woman as her contractions tend to be spaced out and short. In this instance, I recommend slow breathing techniques like the following.

Ujaii breath (Ocean breath)

This is a classic yoga breath, which is very useful throughout labour and wonderful for the early days with a new baby, who loves to hear the calming, deep rhythmic breath of its mother as she holds it close. Begin by sitting in a well supported position. Take a deep inhalation in through the nose, and then breathe out through the mouth as if seeing your breath in front of you on a really cold day. The sound you make is a 'haaaaa' sound, which is soft like a whisper. Breathe this way a few more times, and then as you become more confident, progress to leaving the mouth closed on the exhale. You should still be able to hear an audible sound at the back of the throat (described as sounding like the ocean). Ujaii breath is helpful as it encourages focus and concentration, whilst also bringing a sense of calmness, as the belly rises on the inhale and falls on the exhale.

Counting breath

Establish a deep rhythmic breath, and then silently begin to count the inhale and exhale: Breathing in 1 2 3 4 / Breathing out 1 2 3 4 5 6. The numbers you count don't matter, but ideally the exhale will be longer than the inhale. Even though the mind may wander off many times, it is helpful to keep bringing your attention back to the counting and away from any sensations that you are feeling, which is a great distraction.

Let go breath

Again, once a lovely deep breathing pattern is established, you can begin to inhale and then silently think the word Let, and then as you exhale, you think the word Go. Each time, you can scan down the body from the top of the head to the tips of the toes, softening and relaxing so there is no tension at all.

Golden thread breath

With this breathing technique, you will breathe out through the mouth. Take a deep breath in through the nose to begin, and as you exhale, breathe out a fine stream of air through a small gap that you create between your top lip and bottom lip. As you exhale, you can imagine the fine stream of air as a thin golden thread that carries your attention out into the distance. The purpose of this breath is to slow down the exhalation, which can help to distract the mind. As you breathe and your thoughts travel further and further away from you, you can get lost in the focus. It is described by many women as a useful breathing technique for early labour.

Forceful Breathing Techniques for Established Labour

As the surges intensify, I find that women are more inclined to want to breathe out of their mouths as they exhale, more and more. In this instance, the breath that I find the most successful is one I call dandelion breath. This is a powerful breathing technique that provides the woman with strength and focus. It is also the reason I chose a dandelion symbol for this book and my brand overall, because it can thrive in difficult conditions and has the ability to rise above challenges—a perfect analogy for a woman in labour.

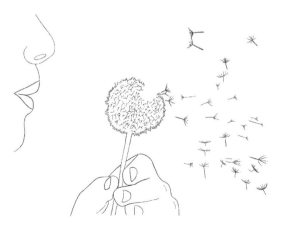

Dandelion breath

Imagine a fluffy-headed dandelion. Take a deep breath in and as you exhale, purse the lips and breathe out fully through the mouth. Your breath should flow out in a steady stream as if blowing towards the dandelion and scattering the seeds far and wide. Each time you exhale, you notice at the end that there is a natural pause. Wait until this is over before taking another long deep breath in and breathing out forcefully, as if you are trying to make a gust of wind.

TENS (Transcutaneous Electrical Nerve Stimulation)

A TENS machine is a battery-operated device that is used to relieve pain and relax muscles. It works by sending electronic stimulation pulses across the surface of the woman's skin and along her nerve strands. This causes the body's own pain killers (endorphins) to be released and reduces the number of pain signals sent to the brain by the spinal cord. This device has four pads that are placed on the woman's mid and lower back, on either side of the spine, four wires that connect to each pad, and a battery-operated box. It has dials to allow its user to turn it up very slowly, providing more stimulation as the labour progresses. The woman is in complete control of the dials, and a maternity TENS, which is different to a normal TENS, has the additional benefit of a boost button that can be pressed at the start and end of each contraction. Lots of feedback suggests that this device can be a welcome distraction—although for some women this can be a negative side effect because for every single contraction, the woman has to remember to press the button to boost the machine, which can bring her back into her thinking brain each and every time. As the birth partner, you can always offer to press the button for her. You can usually tell when a contraction begins and ends by her breathing and movement, although she can also indicate this to you by raising a finger or her hand.

IMPORTANT TO KNOW *For a TENS machine to work effectively, it should be put on in early labour.*

Hypnobirthing

Hypnobirthing is a technique that teaches simple but specific self-hypnosis, through relaxation and breathing methods. By learning to open up the subconscious mind, the woman can reframe her thoughts around her ability to give birth. By entering and then remaining in a calm and relaxed (hypnotic) state, she is more likely to produce high levels of oxytocin and endorphins, thereby resulting in less pain overall. For hypnobirthing to be successful, the woman needs to practise these skills in advance of birth and be familiar with the techniques, as outlined in Chapter 11.

Focal Points and Metaphors

Using a focal point to stare at in labour can be really helpful for some women. It can be simple, like a scan photo, a holiday snap, or words on paper that remind her to 'breathe' or 'relax'. Some women like to write out positive affirmations like 'I am strong' or 'I trust my body', and decorate them in preparation for birth. These ideas can help her to develop a trust and belief in her ability to give birth on the day, which is, of course, better than the fear-based alternatives such as constant doubt and questions about progress. Some women like to take their minds to faraway places through visualisation—for example, walking on the beach with the waves lapping at her feet as each 'wave' of her contraction begins, and then slowly drifting back out as the sensation diminishes. Pam England, a former nurse-midwife, uses an image of a labyrinth as a metaphor for the journey through labour and birth, which works really well for some of my more right-brained clients. She points out that, unlike a maze, a labyrinth has only one way in and one way out. You cannot get lost, or take a wrong turn, as the

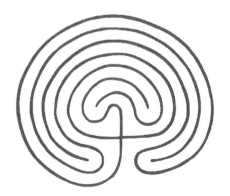

path leads directly to the centre where the woman will meet her baby. It helps women learn to trust the process that the body goes through, and understand that if she were to close her eyes, and keep putting one foot in front of the other, she would reach the middle at her own pace and timing that is right for her and her baby.

Stress Balls

In the book *Birth Skills* by Juju Sundin and Sarah Murdoch, you will find a technique that I have witnessed being used several times over the years to great success. By holding stress balls in each hand and using one of many simple techniques, a woman can divert her attention from the sensation of the contraction and produce endorphins at the same time. This works well for women who do not like passive relaxation techniques. If the woman you are supporting struggles to release tension, and her hands clench up in fear, this will result in more focus on the pain. If energy is present due to the arrival of adrenaline, then this technique can make the most of that extra energy by allowing her to use it in a different way. The woman can squeeze and release the stress balls, finding a rhythm that suits her best. In early labour, squeezing each ball works well, but as labour progresses, most women begin to actually bring the balls together. They start off by tapping them, and then move on as the surges intensify, eventually banging them together quite forcefully. This gives them something very powerful for their arms and hands to do. The book states 'You need to overload your sensory systems with non-painful stimuli to override the uterine pain signal in the brain. Your brain should then register the stress ball activity and not the pain'. Stress balls should be of soft resistance, not hard like tennis balls, and can be coloured for extra visual focus. Some women will also make sounds as they bring the balls together in a repetitive way. The woman could also choose to use other items that provide sensory stimulation like amethyst rocks, squeeze toys, balls with bells or lights, play dough or clay.

Tips for the birth partner include the following.

* Make sure the balls are packed in the birth bag.
* While she is banging the balls, remind her to 'focus on the bang' or 'listen to the bang'.
* Encourage her to focus on the colour.
* Encourage her to coordinate the bangs to the contractions.
* Help her relax her hands and release the balls when each contraction has ended.
* If she is tired, do it for her, and get her to watch you bang the balls together as her focal point.

Complementary Therapies

Many of my clients have used complementary therapies with great success over the years. The woman you are supporting may have a strong preference for one over others, so that is the one you should learn most about, as all of these can be administered by a birth partner.

Homeopathy

The fundamental principle of homeopathy is that it cures 'like with like' by stimulating the body's own natural healing capacity. Each remedy, made from plants and minerals, is highly diluted, ensuring that they are completely safe to use in pregnancy with no side effects at all. During labour, you would choose a remedy to give the woman based on the physical, mental and emotional symptoms she is experiencing. Companies like Helios and Ainsworths sell kits that contain the perfect remedies for pregnancy, labour and birth. There may also be a local homeopath who could provide the woman with a specialised kit that is tailored to her specific needs. Each kit should come with instructions for you to follow on what to use and why.

I am not a homeopath, but these are some of the typical remedies I have in my kit.

- Arnica 200, for bruising and tissue damage in both mother and baby.
- Aconite 200, for fear, pain, shock and panic.
- Pulsatilla 200, for vulnerability, helplessness, feeling let down or tearful.
- Sepia 200, for any woman who feels exhausted or irritable.
- Belladonna 200, if she has a sudden rise in temperature.
- Kali Carb 200, if she feels most of her contractions in her back rather than the front.

Remedies, given mainly in tablet form, can be taken frequently, as often as every 20 minutes and changed as necessary. As labour develops, offer a single remedy when required, and give the minimum dose, stopping as soon as you see progress.

Acupressure Points

Acupressure is the lesser-known companion to acupuncture, but instead of needles, it requires physical pressure. For a labouring woman, accessing certain pressure points (like LI 4, between the thumb and forefinger) can reduce pain, increase blood flow to the uterus, influence hormonal responses and stimulate uterine contractions. There are plenty of free resources online regarding how to find acupressure points, and when to use them in labour. Take time to look them up and make sure you know which acupressure points are safe so you only use them when appropriate.

Aromatherapy

Essential oils are proven to be a safe and effective way to relieve pain in labour, as they are thought to lower cortisol levels in the brain. Many MLUs are equipped with diffusers, and some of the midwives who work within the MLU are trained to blend oils to suit the emotional needs of the women in their care. As my clients usually buy their own remedies that they would like to use, I personally only need to carry a good quality first aid remedy.

For me, lavender is the best, because it is a good all rounder, and helps to keep everyone in the room relaxed and calm. I can place a few drops on a piece of tissue or cotton ball, and leave it close to her, or alternatively I can waft it under her nose if she needs a confidence boost. I can also place a few drops of it into a carrier oil or cream (as it cannot be applied directly onto the skin), and use it to give her a relaxing massage as it is great for muscle tension or aches. If she is interested in using aromatherapy during labour, look up what essential oils are suitable and decide between you if there are any you think she might like to have available. Some essential oils, like Clary Sage, for example, are perfectly safe to use during labour, but are contraindicated for use during pregnancy, so encourage her to research carefully before choosing which ones to buy.

IMPORTANT TO KNOW *Don't put an essential oil on something that cannot be removed from the room. If she decides she doesn't like the smell, you can flush it down the toilet, as even a familiar scent can make her feel nauseous in labour. Also, make sure you keep homeopathy and essential oils away from each other, as the strong smell of aromatherapy oils can cancel out the potency of a homeopathic remedy.*

Reflexology

Similar to acupuncture, reflexology works on acupressure points in the feet. Attending appointments with an experienced reflexologist will be relaxing and very beneficial in pregnancy, preparing the woman and her body for an optimal labour and birth. You can also research where the pressure points are in the feet that support her in labour if necessary, including Spleen 6—just above the ankle bone—which is useful in the event that labour stops.

Gas and Air

Gas and air (Entonox) is a mixture of two gases: 50% nitrous oxide and 50% oxygen. The user breathes in, typically through a plastic mouthpiece.

It can take about 20 seconds to become effective, so a labouring woman is advised to begin breathing in deeply at the start of a contraction, so that by the time she reaches the peak, it will be working. It doesn't take away the sensations, but simply knocks the woman out of her thinking brain and helps her by making her feel a bit sleepy, so she therefore notices them less. It can also make her feel lightheaded and perhaps a bit giggly or 'spaced out'. Gas and air is really helpful to any woman who is feeling anxious, or whose breath is shallow, as it will help her to regulate and deepen her breathing, but it does come with a small word of warning: A woman who uses it too much can become so 'out of it', that she might forget what she is trying to achieve. In some cases, I have seen the woman become upset and cross, and the best way I can describe this is that she feels disillusioned with her labour, and no longer cares about following her plan, so her birth can take a turn in a different direction.

Here are my tips for a birth partner who is supporting a woman using gas and air.

* Side effects can include dizziness, nausea and a dry mouth, so you should give her sips of water after every contraction if you can. I also recommend using a lip balm on her lips to prevent them from drying out and cracking.

* Notice when the contraction is ending and offer to take the handle of the gas and air mouthpiece to hold for her. You can then encourage her to soften and relax all her muscles, as she is usually, by this point, very high. As the effects of the gas begin to wear off, she should slowly start to feel normal again. When the next contraction begins, give her back the handle of the gas, or help to place the mouthpiece in her mouth so that she can breathe deeply again. This is not about you controlling how much gas she has during a contraction; this is to make sure she doesn't use the gas and air in between them. During the break, she should focus on releasing all tension in her body.

- If at any point during labour a decision needs to be made, help her come out of her zoned-out state by recommending that she breathes without using gas and air for the next contraction. This allows for the effects to have a chance to wear off, and she will be able to hear and take part in any discussion regarding her care.

- Continuing the use of gas and air during the pushing phase can sometimes slow down any progress, as the woman is not able to push as well as she might if she didn't have the mouthpiece in. It is very individual to each woman, but worth remembering, so if you think the gas and air is hindering her at this point, encourage her to try a few pushes without using gas and air at the same time.

- Gas and air is available to women at a home birth, brought to the home in small canisters. There may be a restriction as to how many each woman can use. Otherwise, in a labour ward or MLU, it is available on demand. In the event that you attend an induction, it is unlikely that gas and air will be available until the woman leaves the induction bay and is admitted to a labour room, but you can always ask.

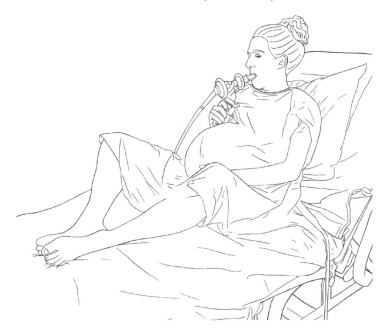

Water Birth

A water birth is where a labouring woman is able to sit or lie in a birthing pool, similar to a large bathtub. The deep water is warm and relaxing and provides a good level of pain relief, as it covers her belly and gives her the freedom to move around weightlessly. She can remain in the pool until the baby is born if she chooses too, as long as the temperature remains around 37 degrees, which is optimal for the baby.

Using a birthing pool can help a woman feel a sense of privacy, as it is easier to maintain physical boundaries, which in turn helps her with positive control. Even though water birth became popular in the 1980s and 90s, it was slow to take off in some hospitals, with midwives lacking the confidence needed to offer the service. As I write in 2020, some hospitals still have incredibly low water birth rates. To my knowledge most have at least one birthing pool, and a local MLU will usually have access to two or three. If the woman you are supporting is hoping to use water in labour, then I recommend choosing an MLU over and above a hospital labour ward. If, however, this is the only option available, then ask for the pool room as soon as you call the hospital to tell them you are coming in, and, assuming there is not already someone else using the pool room, they might save it for you. Often they may even begin filling the pool in preparation for your arrival. Of course, the only guaranteed way to plan a water birth is to give birth at home with the mother buying or renting an inflatable birth pool. Companies like 'Birth Pool in a Box' will sell a complete package including the pool, liner, hose and pumps, and ship it out for next day delivery. You might also find that a doula or friend has one you can hire or borrow, so ask around.

Pethidine

Pethidine is an opioid (like morphine) that is injected into the thigh to help a labouring woman to feel more relaxed and to relieve pain. It has become a familiar option for pain relief, because—as Beverley Beech from

AIMS points out—it is the only pharmacological narcotic that midwives are licensed to prescribe. Pethidine can take about 20 minutes to work, and typically lasts about three to four hours. Unlike other drugs, it doesn't slow labour down, and it can be useful in helping the woman relax and sleep. This is particularly beneficial if she is experiencing a long latent phase (see Chapter 5). Some of the women I know who used this drug in early labour have shared that taking pethidine helped them to get 'out of their head and into their body', which of course is very good for oxytocin production. Some women, however, share negative effects of pethidine, saying they had the odd sensation of being trapped in their own bodies, with nothing to do but wait for it to wear off. Pethidine acts as a muscle relaxant, which also has an effect on the woman's pelvic floor muscles, negatively impacting her ability to push. It is also known to cross the placenta and can cause the baby to become drowsy. This means that if the baby is born before the effects have worn off, he or she can have difficulty breathing and may struggle to feed for several hours or even days after the birth. Pethidine can also make a woman feel nauseous so is often given along with an anti-nausea drug. Some hospitals may use an alternative opioid drug instead such as diamorphine, meptid or remifentanyl, which have similar side effects.

Epidural

An epidural is considered to be the ultimate pain relief, as it can provide a complete block to the woman. It numbs the nerves that carry the pain impulses from the birth canal. It is a type of anaesthetic, and it can only be administered in a main hospital on a labour ward by an anaesthetist. The baby's heart rate will need to be monitored throughout the remainder of the labour once an epidural is sited, and the woman will need to remain on the bed as her legs will slowly become numb. She should be able to lie on her side if the midwife is able to get a good trace on the baby's heartbeat. She will need to have a cannula placed in her hand or arm so that doctors can easily put fluids through. In many hospitals, the woman has overall control of topping up the epidural via a button attached to the machine.

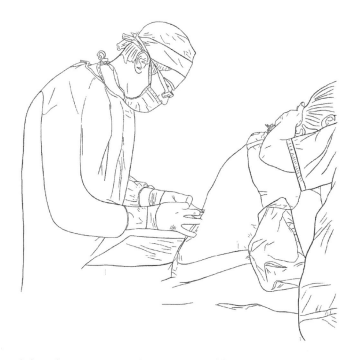

Whilst a big pro is complete pain relief for most women, here are some cons that you as the birth partner should know about epidurals.

* It takes about 15–20 minutes for a thin plastic tube (catheter) to be placed through a needle in the woman's lower back. The needle will eventually be removed and the catheter will remain in position, administering medication throughout the duration of the labour. The woman will need to sit very still during this time. Once in, it will take about another 20 minutes for the epidural to work to its full effect. This means that, assuming an anaesthetist is available at the time of the request, it will be a minimum of 40 minutes from decision to no pain—but realistically, an average of 1 hour can be expected. Gas and air is useful during this time, and your good calming skills

are essential, as once a woman has decided to have an epidural, her tolerance levels for pain are low.

- She is unlikely to be able to eat or drink from the time that the epidural is sited, due to the higher chance of c-section. I therefore recommend getting a good snack into her before the anaesthetist arrives, if possible.

- For one in eight women, the epidural will not work. If that is the case, let the midwife or anaesthetist know as they may be able to help. Sometimes one side of the body experiences more numbness than the other, so in this instance a change in position can help, and the midwife will advise you.

- A common side effect is that the woman's blood pressure may drop, so the doctor is likely to give her IV fluids to help prevent this. She can also suffer with itching, and can feel very shaky.

- Sometimes her legs can become restless, numb or tingly, as the medication begins to take effect. It may last a few hours and again can occur on one side more than another. I recommend rubbing or massaging her legs if she is uncomfortable, to relieve the sensitivity she is experiencing.

- In some cases, an epidural can slow labour down, possibly due to the effects that the drug has on hormone production. If the contractions diminish, breaking the woman's waters or administering a synthetic oxytocin drip may be recommended to help speed up the labour.

- A midwife is likely to remain with you most of the time, due to increased risk, more monitoring, and frequent assessment of pain. It can be quite distracting for you both, as once the woman is pain free, she may find herself chatting with everyone when she should be resting. In this instance, consider turning the lights down, and encourage her not to engage once the epidural is working well, so she can get some sleep before she is expected to begin pushing. Ear plugs and an eye mask are useful at this point.

- The midwife will expect to perform a VE once every four hours. Even if a woman is nine cm dilated at her last examination, she may be expected to wait another four hours before she is checked again. Once full dilation has been established, the midwife will leave her for at least another hour or more to allow for descent of the baby.
- A catheter (a thin plastic tube) may be inserted into the woman's bladder as she will be unable to use the bathroom. It is usually removed shortly after the baby is born.
- There is a 50% likelihood of requiring assistance via ventouse or forceps, which may lead to an episiotomy. This is because a woman cannot feel an urge to push and is more likely to be lying on her back. To try to avoid this, some women leave the epidural to wear off a little until they feel the sensations return, and they can then try pushing whilst lying on their side.
- Epidurals are often a combination of anaesthetics and opioid analgesics. This can increase the chances of the baby having a temporary change in heart rate, trouble breathing, drowsiness and reduced muscle tone, and it may initially make it trickier for the baby to latch on and breastfeed.
- One percent of women will suffer with a headache afterwards. This can usually be treated; you should encourage her to mention it to the midwife.
- Unfortunately, in some situations, a woman who is desperate for an epidural may be told that it is not possible at that time. This is usually because either the anaesthetist is already busy in theatre (in which case, it's worth a try to speak to a more senior midwife and ask if they can access another doctor from a different department in the hospital) or because the woman's labour has progressed quickly and it is deemed 'too late'. This can feel very traumatic for the woman, and she will benefit from your calm support until an anaesthetist becomes available or the baby is born.

IMPORTANT TO KNOW *Despite the list of potential complications, an epidural does give great relief for those women who are really struggling with the intensity of labour. Whilst it is essential to be aware of the side effects and the changes that it may bring to the path her labour is following, the decision to move forward with an epidural will always be the right one, if the woman is deciding for herself.*

QUICK RECAP

Here are the main things to remember when discussing birth management.

- **Discuss all pain relief options.** Talk to her about her thoughts on pain relief options. Ensure that she understands what she wants in regard to her dream birth scenario.

- **What is available?** Make sure she has checked that what she wants to use is available in the location where she has chosen to give birth.

- **What does she need to learn?** If she would like to use more natural birth management techniques, then encourage her to sign up to attend classes and courses like pregnancy yoga and hypnobirthing to give her the knowledge and tools she will need.

- **Complementary therapies.** If she wants to use a complementary therapy during labour, you will need to know and fully understand when to use them and how.

- **Safety Word.** Remind her that if she has decided to have a safety word in place, you will continue to encourage her to keep going during labour at all times unless she safety words you.

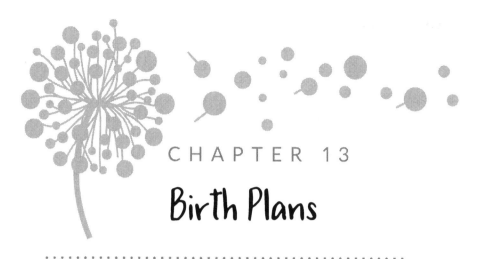

CHAPTER 13

Birth Plans

The power of a birth plan isn't the actual plan; it's the process of becoming educated about all of your options.

A birth plan is a set of preferences that a woman has decided on that includes everything she needs to convey to her care providers. The making of this list is something you should both discuss in detail, and when it is completed, you will have a valuable tool to use on the day of the birth. There is great power in writing out a birth plan and exploring the idea that this is her birth, not her care providers', so she should take ownership of the decisions made. The way the birth plan—and the individual preferences it includes—are worded will help ensure that her wishes are easily understood and respected where possible. There should also be an underlying element of flexibility towards those aspects she cannot control. For example, if she wants a water birth and there is only one pool at the hospital she has chosen, there is always the possibility that someone else might be using it already.

How Relevant is a Birth Plan?

It is common for my clients to question the relevance of a birth plan. They are often told by their friends not to bother writing one, as 'birth plans are a joke!' It is fair to admit that around the turn of this century, birth plans had a bad name, and were definitely considered to be a waste of time as they seemed to set any couple who wrote one up for failure. Most would look back at their birth plan and say that they didn't achieve any of the items written on it, with some admitting they didn't even get it out of the bag. They may have become educated about what to write on their plan, but have not learned enough information to be able to advocate for themselves during pregnancy, or on the day. So when their dream birth went out the window, it was easy to blame themselves, believing they were foolish to have wanted an easy experience and that it had been ridiculous to have a birth plan in the first place.

In my classes, I make sure that couples understand the value of having their own set of guidelines. They are important because the pregnant woman is able to sit down with her birth partner and share information about her 'Plan A'; look at all locations and options for birth management; talk about decision making; explore positive and negative control; choose a safety word; and discuss 'Plan B', including what would happen in the event of an induction or c-section. The birth plan is also important because, as the birth partner, you then have a document which helps you to remember and understand what is important to her. This is a resource you can refer to and share with anyone that provides care for her during the birth, especially if there is a change of shift. It is important that she writes a birth plan that is sensible and easy to read, so that you can ensure her preferences are voiced and met with respect.

Documenting Her Preferences

The last few years have seen birth plans become more widely accepted by medical professionals, and there are now some amazing resources online with novel ideas about how to document her preferences, including using pictures and diagrams. The list must be clear, so that you are able to use it to support her choices on the day without disturbing her. It becomes the first point of reference if any initial decisions need to be made, so make sure that she only writes down the items that are relevant to her chosen venue and are achievable by her care provider. There is always the option of writing a birth plan for Plan A and a separate one for Plan B. I find the plan particularly useful when the woman has vocally indicated she wants to avoid something and the midwife overlooks this preference or wants her to reconsider. For example: Let's say that one of her preferences states that she would like to leave the cord to finish pulsating. Then, in the early post-natal period, when you are both happily gazing at the baby, you notice the midwife getting ready to clamp the cord. At this point, you would be able to remind the midwife that the preferences state that she wants to leave the cord to carry on pulsating and 'wait for white' by saying something like 'STOP! It says on the birth plan that she wants to leave the cord alone'. You might even say to the woman, 'Is that still the case?' This encourages the midwife to hold off and wait a while longer.

Birth Plan Checklist

This checklist can serve as a discussion guide for you to go through with her, and is available as a free download with the purchase of this book.

1. Philosophy of Birth

What does your ideal birth look like? What do you want to achieve? What do you both need to learn and read in order to understand how to achieve your ideal birth? What classes do you need to sign up for to boost your understanding of the decisions you may be expected to make during labour and birth?

2. Hospital Guidelines and Policies

Where can you give birth in your area: home, midwife-led or obstetric-led care? What facilities are available to choose from in each of these locations? Are you low risk or high risk? Do you understand the guidelines and policies at your local unit that may affect you? The NICE intrapartum guidelines may help you understand any recommendations given; see their website at nice.org.uk, or ask your midwife for information, as policies do vary. What are your views on student observation? Monitoring? VEs? Induction? Pain relief? C-section? Do you know the pros and the cons of each in order to make a well informed decision?

3. Environment

What surroundings might affect you? Do you both know how to adjust your environment during labour? What will you want to take with you that will make you feel more at ease? (This category can include preferences on music, positioning, props, smells, gadgets, snacks, or breathing techniques).

4. Plan B

Sometimes plans change. Ensure you understand what you would want to happen if you had to change course. What is your Plan B? If you had to go to theatre, would your partner come with you? Do you know and understand what options you have if a c-section becomes necessary? If the baby had to go to special care, who would go with the baby?

5. After Care/Umbilical Cord and Placenta

The decisions aren't over once your baby is born (see Chapter 16). Do you want to be the first person to touch the baby? Do you want the baby placed straight onto your skin? Do you understand the choices that can be made about the umbilical cord? Do you want an injection to expel the placenta, or do you want the placenta to come away on its own? Do you know what checks will be done to you? Do you know what checks will be done to the baby? Do you know why Vitamin K is recommended?

6. Feeding Your Baby

The baby may want to feed within the first few hours after birth. Have you decided how you want to feed your baby? If you intend to breastfeed, are you aware of the support in your area? Do you understand supply and demand? Do you know how many times a newborn baby feeds? Do you know what a tongue tie is? Are you aware of the common issues mothers face when learning to breastfeed? Do you have information on how to hand express or use a breast pump?

7. Putting a Plan Together

Once she has considered the questions above, she can begin to put her preferences down on paper. I recommend a simple list that can be read quickly and easily. Be specific and don't add information that is not relevant. Please keep flexibility in mind.

> **REMEMBER**
> A birth plan is not a legal document but simply a communication tool.

ALICE'S STORY Alice had been planning a home birth and had been discussing it with her midwives but felt unsupported. In desperation, she eventually hired me as her doula at 37 weeks. She told me that she felt that her relationship with the midwives had broken down and she was unsure what to do. She gave me permission to meet with them on her behalf to look at ways to restore trust. At that meeting, the two midwives admitted that they couldn't understand why she had felt the need to employ a doula. They told me that they had been very supportive of her wishes and even had her 4-page birth plan on the wall in their office for all the midwives to read in case they were on call the night of her birth. 'Wait!' I said in disbelief. 'She wrote a birth plan covering four sides of A4 paper and you didn't see that as a red flag?' Writing out all that information was a clear sign to me that she lacked trust in the midwives' ability to help her achieve her dream birth, and she was trying to get them to listen to her by flooding them with her wishes. Fortunately, after the meeting, I was able to help re-build the relationship Alice had with the local midwives. Then, together, we narrowed down her preferences to a specific list, highlighting what was most important to her in an easy-to-understand format. Alice felt that she was back in control of her birth and could trust that those around her would support everything that she hoped for. A few days later, she had a beautiful home birth, which went exactly the way that she had wanted. This was her final birth plan:

Alice's Birth Preferences

Safety word: Alabama

- Please do not perform any procedure without my consent.
- Pain relief is not to be offered unless requested.
- I am trying to achieve a calm, quiet, positive environment.
- I would like limited monitoring.
- I would like the umbilical cord to be white and empty before it is cut.
- I would like immediate skin-to-skin with the baby and am planning to breastfeed.

• •

In reality, no one should need to write more than a handful of bullet points to express her preferences. In my experience, midwives really want to help women achieve their dream birth, so will work closely with women and their birth partners to ensure that everything goes well. However, the midwife is unlikely to have time to read lengthy sentences that explain the woman's thoughts and wishes in great detail.

In preparation for this book, I searched through my files of previous clients' birth plans. Whilst no two women that I support are the same, there was a big similarity in the way they wrote their birth preferences. Here, I have included some examples of ones that work well, and also some that don't. These examples are all shared from real clients who have given permission for their use.

Writing an Ineffective Birth Plan

Sample 1: Deborah's Birth Wishes

Dear Midwife,

It took a very long time for us to conceive this child, and we are keen to make sure that the birth goes really well and exactly how we are planning. We want a completely natural birth and I want the room to be set up nicely with a calm, relaxing atmosphere and music. I am definitely going to use the birth pool for pain relief and will probably go on to deliver in there too. I understand that pain relief will interfere with the birth and so I want to state from the outset that I do not want to be offered any pain relief at all, except gas and air. My birthing partners (the father of the baby and my mother) will be with me at all times. I would like to avoid any students being present at the birth as I have had a bad experience in the past, so would not feel comfortable with them taking over any aspect of my care. I am having a natural third stage and my husband will cut the cord. He can get a bit emotional so will need to be watched carefully. I would also really like him to have some skin-to-skin time with the baby after the birth, but he isn't keen on that. I am really unsure about the pros and cons of Vitamin K, so would appreciate your help in working out if we would like the baby to receive it or not. I want to book a private room and as I intend to breastfeed, I would like to stay in hospital until my milk flow is regulated and established.

Top Tip: Don't waffle.

There is no need for the birth plan to talk about issues that have no relevance to the people caring for her. The midwife, in this example, would need to get a highlighter pen to identify exactly what this woman is looking for.

Sample 2: Tanya's Birth Plan

1. I refuse pethidine.

2. I am going to remain upright throughout.

3. I am having a natural third stage.

4. I only want a midwife in the room when I ask for one.

5. I want a private room.

Top Tip: Don't be too rigid or rude.

This gives an air of superiority which would instantly put your relationship with the midwife on the wrong foot—not a good start! There is also no benefit to writing something that has no flexibility or any allowance for the woman to change her own mind. Tanya's midwife will probably be scared to attend this labour.

Writing an Effective Birth Plan

All of the client samples that follow are birth plan ideas that show the woman's preferences in short, clear and specific bullet points, with a degree of flexibility. In my opinion, there is no benefit to being overly polite, so try not to constantly use words like 'please' or 'can I have'. Remember that a woman can write more than one birth plan, and she can change her mind regarding her preferences at any point during labour and birth. Sample 6 shows a caesarean plan in case the woman you're supporting would like to write one to have ready. In this instance, you should leave it in the birth bag and only get it out if required.

Sample 3: Jayne's Birth Preferences

1. I am happy to go with the flow, but would like to remain upright for as much of the birth as possible.

2. I am open to pain relief, and my preference, when required, would be to try the birthing pool and gas and air before an epidural.

3. It's very important to me to be skin-to-skin with the baby as soon as she is born.

4. I am having my placenta encapsulated after the birth and would like to ensure it is stored correctly once it has been examined.

5. My baby will be having oral Vitamin K.

Sample 4: Laura's Birth Preferences

Yes, Please:

- Use the pool if it is available
- Gas and air and epidural will be considered
- Delay cord clamping, unless medical reason not to
- Immediate skin to skin

No, Thanks:

- Talking, especially during a contraction
- Electronic Fetal Monitoring (unless necessary)
- Routine Vaginal Examinations

Sample 5: Katie's Birth Preferences

General

- Hypnobirthing: Quiet and dimly lit environment. Any discussion have first outside the birth room.

- Pain relief: Do not offer me pain relief. I am aware of what is available and will ask if required.

- Vaginal examinations: Only at our request, please.

- Monitoring: Happy to be monitored routinely by Doppler (no need to ask permission each time).

- Do not discuss time / timings in the birth room.

The Birth

- No coached pushing (I only want to push when I feel the urge).

- I would like to catch the baby.

- We would like to discover the gender of the baby ourselves.

- Allow as long as possible before cutting the cord (wait for white).

- Dad would like to cut the cord.

Third Stage / Afterwards

- Physiological third stage; no Syntometrine injection unless bleeding heavily.

- Placenta: We would like to keep our placenta.

- First hour: Skin to skin immediately. Baby to remain unclothed and any weighing or measurements to be delayed for the first hour.

- Feeding: We wish to breastfeed and would like this to begin naturally.

- Vitamin K: Injection please.

Sample 6: Thea's Caesarean Birth Preferences

I would like my partner to be with me at all times.

I would like to be communicated with as much as possible and to be kept informed of what is happening.

I would like the screen to be lowered at the point that the baby is being born so I can see as much as possible.

I would like immediate skin to skin with the baby—this is very important to me.

I would like to allow the cord to pulsate for as long as possible. Please discuss this with me before clamping or cutting.

Introducing the Birth Plan

As the birth partner, it is your job to present the birth plan to the midwife or doctor at the point when they become involved in her care during labour. She may have already shown a copy to her midwife or doctor in the antenatal period, but the same person is unlikely to be involved in her care on the day. It is important to have several copies to hand out, ideally on one single sheet of paper, and not placed inside a file or a bag. Leave it somewhere in the room, so it can be accessed easily by the midwives or doctors and make sure you have a copy handy for yourself.

Home Birth

Ideally, you will greet the midwives at the door of the home, and show them into a room that is not the one where the woman is labouring. Consider which room she might give birth in, thinking about the layout of her home, and see if there is a space to accommodate the midwives in their own private area close by. This will enable the midwives to settle themselves into the house, take off their coats, and bring themselves down to your peaceful calm level. They will have space to lay out their equipment and write their notes where there is plenty of light. Before taking the midwife in to meet the woman, give them the list of her preferences and ask them to let you know if they have any questions. You can also take this time to fill them in on any information you want to share about the labour so far, always remembering to use a low, quiet voice if possible. When you are ready to invite them into the room where the woman is labouring, you can ask them to follow you in quietly and introduce themselves, and to help you carry out her preferences.

MLU/Hospital

Upon arrival at the unit, you will either go straight to a desk or be greeted by a midwife at the door. If the woman has handheld notes, you can make sure that the birth plan is stapled to the front, so it will be the first thing the midwife sees. If the woman has electronic notes, you can give the midwife who is assigned to look after you a copy of the birth plan when they show you into the room or cubicle. If there are shift changes during the time you are at the hospital, you can ask the new midwives if they have read the birth plan. In some cases, if a client prefers not to print her birth plan, you can send a virtual pdf copy direct to the midwife's mobile phone. When labour happens quickly, there may be no time for the midwife to read the list. In this instance, you might have to get the woman's preferences across verbally.

Changing the Birth Plan

At any time, regardless of why, if a woman 'safety words' you, then you are switching to Plan B. Her right to change her birth plan is not something that you need to discuss other than how you can help her identify what she would like to do next. It is not uncommon, however, for the midwife to be the one who makes a recommendation that involves a change to the woman's birth preferences. This could be during labour itself, or after the baby is born. For example, if the woman has specified that she does not want a vaginal examination, but many hours have passed with no signs of progress, then the midwife or doctor might want to talk to her about this. They may explain that as time has gone by with no sign of a shift into second stage, they would like to assess her to see what is happening and check the baby's position. In Chapter 14, I have provided you with a useful tool that uses the acronym T-BRAIN, to ask a series of questions when making medical decisions. It is important to use this to ask questions you feel apply in this kind of scenario, to ensure that a well informed decision is made. Also bear in mind that birth preferences are not set in stone. If the woman wants to accept a recommendation and therefore move on from her original preferences, it is perfectly acceptable for her to do so, but if she hasn't then she can continue to decline. Have a discussion with her around how she would like to proceed and ask the midwife or doctor to leave the room, if necessary, giving you time to talk in private.

· ·

STEPH'S STORY During Steph's labour, a doctor walked into the room after having a discussion with the midwife outside about her. He had apparently made the decision without ever meeting Steph and her partner that her labour was slow to progress (probably compared to the other women on the labour ward at that time) and that it would be in everyone's best interests if she had a c-section. When the doctor introduced himself, he simply said " Hello, I'm Dr So-and-so, and I have just been speaking to the midwife outside. We think it's time to get this baby out, don't you?" Steph was shocked as she had not seen this coming. She had not been told that the midwife was going outside to speak to the doctor. She became very upset that they didn't feel she was progressing, as she had been coping so well. Yes, she was tired and had been in labour for almost 2 days, but she was really keen to avoid a c-section and have a natural birth. In that moment, her partner was able to use the T-BRAIN tool (see Chapter 14), and after asking some questions to gain more information regarding the advice given, she was able to confidently ask the doctor, 'Can we wait one more hour?' The doctor said 'of course' and strode out of the room. Steph and her partner, again, gave each other shocked looks and praised themselves for buying more time. They were then able to chat about how they felt, discuss the options that were available, and admit that the labour was in fact not progressing. This was something that they had avoided talking about up to that point. In the end, about 45 minutes later, they themselves decided to go and tell the midwife that they felt a c-section was appropriate and they would like to go ahead. Because Steph had some control over that situation, with the help of her birth partner, she always felt her birth was a wonderful experience and never regretted the decisions she made.

. . . .

Coercion

Coercion (noun)

The use of force or intimidation to gain compliance.

This is a tough subject to write about, but unfortunately, I have witnessed coercive behaviour many times over the last 20 years. I have also heard about it far too many times via other doulas and online social media groups. Even so, I still struggle to admit to my clients that it exists. My old romantic, dreamy heart wants to believe that no one would ever want to force or threaten a woman to change her preferences in pregnancy or during labour because it suits the bureaucracy of the hospital more than the woman or the baby. I want to believe that a medical professional who is speaking to a woman and her partner would never use coercive language, but I know that it is happening. What I don't know is if the midwife or doctor themselves are aware that their words are perceived as coercive by the recipient. So I want to start by looking at ways that it can happen, so you have the ability to spot it for yourself, in case you and the woman you are supporting are on the receiving end of coercive behaviour.

First, there are the obvious examples to spot, such as a male doctor suggesting: 'If you were my wife, I would be telling you to . . . .'. Or any doctor saying 'I wouldn't want it on my conscience if anything were to happen to your baby'. But then there are the subtle comments from any care providers like 'hop on the bed and I'll examine you', or 'I'm just going to put a cannula in your hand so we can give you some fluids'.

Any sentences that begin with:

* 'Hi, I have just come to...'
* 'I am just going to...'
* 'Can you just...'
* 'First I need to...
* 'I'm afraid I cannot do that if you are not prepared for me to...'
* 'You won't be allowed if I can't...'
* 'So what we will do now is...'
* 'But you are so tired, just let me..."

You can insert any of these phrases to finish the sentence: book you in for induction, examine you, break your waters, listen to your baby, take a blood sample, get you out of the pool, set up a syntocinon drip, give you some antibiotics. These words may sound reasonably harmless, but if a woman is directed without discussion, the woman effectively has no opportunity to give her informed consent. It is being assumed by the caregiver that the woman will comply, even when she has not been given knowledge of the risks and benefits. In my experience, most women are more than happy to accept a procedure or take the advice given by her midwife or doctor. The caregivers, however, should not just assume that the woman doesn't need to be included in any decision being made about her care. As the birth partner, you should ask questions that will guide both of you if you find yourself in this situation.

> Any comment, statement or instruction that does not follow a discussion about consent, is therefore not consent.

Human Rights in Childbirth

Birthrights is an organisation set up in 2013 by human rights barrister Elizabeth Prochaska and Rebecca Schiller, a doula and author. Their aim is to provide advice and information about human rights in childbirth to women, doctors and midwives, and to campaign for respectful and safe maternity care that protects a woman's fundamental rights. I have met them both on their travels around the country and I have listened to them speak at various conferences. I've witnessed the excellent training given to midwives and doctors, that teaches them how to document the information they provide to women and their partners, ensuring all medical professionals are able to accurately record the decisions that women in their care make, thereby eliminating the possibility of litigation.

A recent court case demonstrated a need for such training. The BMJ (formerly the *British Medical Journal*) wrote:

The Montgomery v Lanarkshire case of March 2015 drew fresh attention to informed consent. Nadine Montgomery, a woman with diabetes and of small stature, delivered her son vaginally; he experienced complications owing to shoulder dystocia, resulting in hypoxic insult with consequent cerebral palsy. Her obstetrician had not disclosed the increased risk of this complication in vaginal delivery, despite Montgomery asking if the baby's size was a potential problem. Montgomery sued for negligence, arguing that, if she had known of the increased risk, she would have requested a caesarean section. The Supreme Court of the UK announced judgment in her favour in March 2015. The ruling overturned a previous decision by the House of Lords, which had been law since at least the mid 1980s. It established that, rather than being a matter for clinical judgment to be assessed by professional medical opinion, a patient should be told whatever they want to know, not what the doctor thinks they should be told.

Nadine Montgomery, who recently became a patron of Birthrights, wrote her own personal account of the experience on their website: 'I was brought in for induction of labour at 38 weeks, and it was once again noted that I was having a large baby. Oxytocin was administered the next day to augment (begin) contractions. After many hours I started to become unwell with a high temperature, and a decision to take me to theatre for a trial of forceps was made at around 5 pm the following evening. A different doctor brought me a consent form saying 'trial of forceps' and before I signed that I asked this doctor what that meant. I was told that they would be able to assess me properly in theatre where they could see better. If there was room to use forceps then they would attempt that, if not they would resort to a caesarean section. I had no real understanding about the procedure being proposed or the potential complications that could arise'.

Shroud-waving

Shroud-waving (noun)

The practice of focusing on the potentially negative effects of a particular policy in order to influence public opinion.

The reason I shared Nadine Montgomery's account of her experience with you was not to scare you into believing that something can go wrong during the birth you attend, but merely to highlight how individual each person's risk is. In her example, she was a very small woman with a condition that had the potential for her baby to grow bigger than average. I also assume that after being taken to theatre for a trial of forceps, she was likely to be lying on her back, which would have limited space in her pelvis even more. The complication she experienced would not be the same for all women. The *Montgomery v Lanarkshire* case has highlighted the need for doctors and midwives to be more transparent about women's individual circumstances, and help the woman and her partner to understand all options, regardless of the doctor's own opinion. This gives the woman the opportunity to decide for herself what risks she is prepared to accept. In reality, this is not what has been happening. Since 2015, I have witnessed a rise in defensive practice for a woman in a similar scenario who is pregnant with a potential 'big baby'. I hear even more coercion in the form of 'shroud-waving', with women being told that their baby could die if they don't accept a recommended procedure. Instead of doctors and midwives having detailed discussions for each individual woman's circumstances, along with their reasoning for any recommendations offered, they merely make sure that they have said the words 'shoulder dystocia'—a situation where a baby (regardless of size) can get one of its shoulders stuck as it is being born. Once mentioned, suitably filling the parents with fear, they have done their due diligence. The midwife or doctor will then typically go ahead without discussion, and book the woman in for a scan, informing her that she will probably need to have her baby early via an induction. This is despite the fact that research suggests an induction is more likely to result in shoulder dystocia, as was the case for Mrs. Montgomery.

. . . .

GRACE'S STORY Grace was told that she had low PAPP-A (pregnancy-associated plasma protein-A) after a blood screening test was performed early in her pregnancy. The midwife explained that it was a hormone made by the placenta, and a low level could indicate the placenta may not work well leading to an increased chance that the baby could be born early, may have a lower weight, and also that Grace had an increased risk of developing pre-eclampsia. The recommendation for a woman with low PAPP-A is to have regular scans to monitor the baby, and an induction around 40 weeks.

She was now on the high-risk pathway despite being well in her pregnancy overall. Grace did a lot of research and discovered that screening for PAPP-A was relatively new, and that there is little evidence yet to show the benefits of inducing labour versus the risks. Grace was therefore happy to attend the scans and keep a close eye on the baby's growth. The nearer it got to her due date, the more confident she felt about her options, and after weighing up her own personal circumstances, she chose to decline the induction.

Vulnerability

Women are extremely vulnerable during the late stages of pregnancy and are therefore very coercible. So if the woman you are supporting is told during her pregnancy that her baby is too small, her baby is too big, she is too old, she has too much liquor (water around the baby), she has not enough liquor, she has low Papp-A, her BMI is too high, her BMI is too low, her pelvis is small, she has had too many previous pregnancies, her babies are born too close together, she had a previous vaginal tear, she had a previous post-partum haemorrhage, she has low iron, she had a previous c-section—then she is likely to agree to whatever is being recommended. She may be completely unaware that she even has a choice, because her birth has been labelled as 'risky'. If the woman feels intimidated by the doctor or midwife, she may feel too nervous to question them. In this scenario, you can help her by asking for evidence that backs up any medical advice given, and then insist on some time to consider the pros and cons. If this is her first baby, she may be scared and nervous that she isn't qualified to make the right decisions about her care. She may not feel like her instincts are particularly reliable, as she has not tuned into them before. You can help her by reminding her that as long as her decision is well informed, then that is what matters. Research the websites, articles and blogs listed throughout this book, and check out the Resources section at the back.

Risk Assessment

During the pregnancy, many tests are carried out to check the health and well being of the mother and baby. Midwives are under great pressure to 'risk assess' women, and if they don't spot a baby in a breech position or identify a baby who is growing too fast or too slow, and something goes wrong, they can be in a lot of trouble. The litigious nature of modern society does mean that more women will be sent for checks or procedures that might not be necessary, even if they are deemed as being in the interest of safety for her or the baby at the time. The biggest issue with these extra tests, checks or scans, is that they can leave shards of doubt or fear in the woman's mind about her ability to give birth. In this instance, it is more likely that these precautionary measures may influence her to switch to Plan B, even though there was never a problem in the first place. As always, remind her to question the pros and cons of any extra checks advised before she decides to accept.

IMPORTANT TO KNOW   *The midwife will check the growth measurement of the woman's uterus by using a tape measure. This method is not always accurate, and different midwives can get varying results. If the woman has a full bladder, for example, she may get a false reading.*

Survivors of Sexual Abuse

For many survivors of abuse, the journey of pregnancy and birth can be an extremely triggering experience. I wish I could share with you that everyone who cares for such women during this time is respectful, but it is not always the case. The woman you are supporting may or may not have disclosed to you that she is a survivor, so my advice is to always show her a high level of esteem and then you know you are getting it right.

* Language must not be coercive. She should not have to justify when 'no' means 'no'. If you feel that you have to take the midwife or doctor who speaks to you both during the birth process aside to repeat this, then find the confidence to do so.

- Don't use belittling praise, saying things like 'good girl' when she lies still and does what she is told—this can be very triggering for the woman.

- Ask her how she would like examinations to be performed if she decides to have them, with prompting questions like 'would you like the midwife to tell you what is happening at all times?' (You would be amazed at how many doctors and midwives will have a silent rummage around when performing a VE and will 'shush' the woman for complaining).

- She may find it difficult being examined by a male midwife or doctor, so request a female in this instance.

- Speak to her about how she feels about dim light, bright light and being observed by students or other midwives if this is relevant.

- Being covered and clothed may be very important to her. Talk to her about what she would like to wear for her labour and make sure she has plenty of spare clothes.

- Breastfeeding can be difficult for survivors, particularly if their breasts were involved in the abuse they experienced, so bear in mind that if she doesn't want to breastfeed, she doesn't have to justify that to anyone.

QUICK RECAP

Here are the main things to remember when discussing birth plans.

- **Relevancy.** Talk about the relevancy of a birth plan that contains a specific list of her preferences, outlining her thoughts concisely about the type of birth she is hoping to achieve.

- **Birth plan checklist.** Ensure that, before any decisions are made, you work your way through the birth plan checklist so that you are both aware of the issues in question.

- **What are her preferences?** Ask her to write down her preferences. Go through them with her and check that they are clear and simple but also relevant to the birth she is planning.

- **Print several copies of the birth plan.** Have several copies of the birth plan ready to share with the midwife who is supporting the woman on the day of the birth in case there is a shift change.
- **Recognise coercive language.** Understand that language used by care providers during pregnancy and birth can sometimes be coercive.

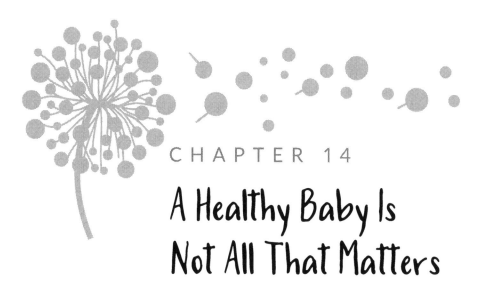

CHAPTER 14

A Healthy Baby Is Not All That Matters

Humanising birth means understanding that the woman giving birth is a human being, not a machine and not just a container for making babies.

–Marsden Wagner

I am sure that almost every pregnant woman would say that her goal is to have a healthy baby, and that a safe birth is important to her. I have no doubt that she would add that during the process, she would like to be treated well, feel loved and respected by all that care for her, and be able to describe her birth as a positive experience. The fact is that, for some, labour doesn't go well, and the woman experiences a long and difficult birth. Her preferences can go out the window, and interventions may take place that leave her feeling like she lost control somewhere along the way. The woman can often feel disappointed and ultimately traumatised by the birth. As the early postnatal days go by, she struggles to comprehend what she has been through, so far removed from the dream birth she had planned. Every time she tries to speak of her experience, she hears the words 'at least you have a healthy baby' from those around her. She may be feeling pretty broken both physically and emotionally whilst coping with extreme exhaustion. There are an abundance of hormones flooding her body, which make her feel elated one minute and have her sobbing the next. During this time, her feelings are overshadowed as she takes care of the baby, which leads her to eventually suppress these emotions, and even she herself begins to think that 'a healthy baby is all that matters'. Her own guilt as the disappointment and exhaustion continue to wash over her lead to an unsatisfying few months with her new baby. She may be unable to describe why this is the case, because she might not recognise that her feelings are related to her birth experience. As a birth partner and therefore potentially a spouse, relative or friend, it is important for you to remind her that she matters too.

The intent of this chapter is to explore ways to help you both understand that, whilst sometimes things don't go to plan, and the woman may experience a difficult birth, it does not need to be a negative experience. Her feelings about what happened to her should not be dumbed down, and ignored, and she should know that even though she now has a baby to look after, it is not acceptable for her needs to be left at the bottom of the pile.

> ## A difficult birth does not need to be a negative experience!

Taking ownership of the birth

A woman has only one opportunity to have each birth experience. There is no dress rehearsal. Whilst each one no doubt shapes the next, some women who have a traumatic birth may stop, choosing not to have more children because the thought of giving birth again is simply too much to consider. The thing is, no woman should have to experience giving birth in a negative way at all. Her caregivers should not ignore her as a human being and forget how equally important her life is, if the labour takes time to progress. She shouldn't have the baby dragged from her body leaving her damaged and in permanent pain. She shouldn't have to suffer other functional issues, and have people excuse it as having been essential to save the baby. In advance of her first birth experience, or any that follow, she needs to understand how to take ownership of her birth and ask you as her birth partner to support her through that process. During my antenatal courses, I teach about this in great detail. I love to say 'You will only have this birth once, so make it the best birth you can', and I explain that the woman and her birth partner have the ability to ask for what they want, both in the antenatal period and during the birth itself. I want everyone to understand that the guidelines set out by their chosen place of birth are not set in stone. I share that they hold the power of a positive birth experience, and I talk about their responsibilities in the birth process. I share that same information with you in this book. I want all birth partners to know that their wives, girlfriends, family members or clients will find birth easier if they know they are the decision maker—'No decision about me, without me', to use the NHS slogan. So please keep that in mind as you read through this chapter, because you are her secret weapon when it comes to achieving a positive birth experience, regardless of what journey the birth takes.

Pulling the Dead Baby Card

Did you know that many women are told that if they don't agree to do what their doctor is telling them their baby could die? It is a common predicament that women find themselves in, whilst sitting in front of a healthcare professional who is trying to coerce them into consenting to an induction, a c-section or similar intervention (see Chapter 13). It is rare to hear a balanced viewpoint during these conversations, and most doctors or midwives will only give women information that persuades them to agree to the recommended procedure. AIMS (Association for Improvements in Maternity Services) writes books and journals that make excellent resources for parents to be. I highly recommend their book *Am I Allowed,* which is essential reading for any pregnant woman and her birth partner.

· ·

DEBBIE'S STORY Debbie met with her doctor, who advised her to have
an induction at no later than 40 weeks due to her maternal age. He told her
that 'remaining pregnant past that point will double your risk of stillbirth,
and you wouldn't want that on your conscience, now, would you?' When
I met her, she was understandably very upset, and she confirmed that the
doctor had not at any time pointed out the risks of induction versus the
risk of remaining pregnant. Giving him the benefit of the doubt, she made
another appointment, which I was able to attend. During that meeting, she
asked him some simple questions which we had agreed upon together, that
enabled her to make a well informed decision about whether to accept the
induction or take her pregnancy forward one day at a time. As an example,
two of the questions were: 'What is the real risk to me regarding stillbirth?'
and 'What alternatives are there if I choose to wait?' He told her that the
risk of stillbirth nationally was 1 in 1,000 babies, but that it increases to 2
in 1,000 babies for women over 40 years old. Originally he simply told her
that the risk doubled, but he didn't put it into context. He acknowledged
that she was fit and healthy, and he admitted that she didn't have to have
an induction if she didn't want one. Moving forward he would offer her
extra scans and monitoring of the baby. She was shocked and amazed at
the difference in the doctor's behaviour when she began to ask appropriate
questions. By bringing herself back into the conversation, she was then able
to make a well informed decision.

· ·

Question Everything

At any stage of pregnancy or during labour and birth, it may become obvious that you as the birth partner need to start asking questions, for your
own benefit and also for the woman you are supporting as she makes decisions about her care. In this instance, you can use the popular acronym
T-BRAIN (see Figure 12.1).

Figure 12.1 T-BRAIN Questions

T	**Time**
	Is there time to discuss options, or is this an emergency?
B	**Benefits**
	What are the benefits to the recommendations given?
R	**Risks**
	Are there any risks involved to mother or baby?
A	**Alternatives**
	Are there any alternatives to consider before making a decision?
I	**Instincts**
	What are the woman's instincts saying?
N	**Nothing**
	If she chooses to wait, can she change her mind at any time?

Feel free to ask one, two or all of the questions in the box, along with others you think of. You will know what questions are relevant at the time based on what you have already been told. The questions you ask should fill in the gaps of your knowledge to give you and the woman you are supporting the information she needs to make an informed decision if necessary.

Making Decisions in Pregnancy

The T-BRAIN tool in this chapter is valuable for any woman and birth partner whose doctor or midwife appears to be discussing a way forward with her care that excludes her from the conversation. By remaining calm and asking questions about all the options, you will bring yourselves back into the discussion. Once your questions have been answered, you can then thank the doctor or midwife and tell them that you will let them know her decision as soon as she is ready. If you find that your questions are not well received, or (for example) the doctor is not listening and becomes insistent on giving the pregnant woman a date for a procedure—like an induction or c-section—when she has already expressed she doesn't want one, it might be easier to accept the booking, smile and leave the room. In my experience, it is pointless continuing a meeting with someone who is not respectful, and it is not worth getting into any further debate. Once you have left, you can then easily go straight to the antenatal clinic reception desk, and cancel the appointment. You can then arrange to change doctors to one who is more open to her preferences. Some women in this situation may even decide to change hospitals if they feel it necessary, by contacting another local hospital and speaking to a senior midwife with the authority to arrange a personalised care plan.

Conflicting Information

One woman I recently spoke to who had a c-section with her first baby was told at an antenatal appointment during her second pregnancy that an induction would be very dangerous for her. Her consultant pointed out that she would not be allowed to have an induction because she had a very high chance of uterine rupture due to having a previous c-section. When she was near 42 weeks and still pregnant, another doctor told her that she would be booked in for an induction the next day. She became hysterical and was confused by what they were saying to her. She told me that she felt they were putting her life in danger by making her have a procedure where she would rupture and die. She didn't realise she had a choice and that she was able to decline the recommendation of an induction. It was not put across to her that this was only one of several options available to her. It was assumed that she would just do what she was told. In this instance, her options were:

- She could decline the induction and attend the hospital regularly for monitoring.
- She could have a discussion about what type of induction was safest for her (see Chapter 15).
- She could choose to have another c-section.

She was not given any information about what options she did have, and what the benefits and risks of each one were. She was not led to believe she had any say in the decision-making process. She was simply told that she was being booked for an induction.

Making Decisions in Labour

If the woman you are supporting is in active labour, and at any point it becomes obvious that a decision has to be made, use the T-BRAIN tool as much as you need to. Once your questions have been asked, you can then ask the midwife or doctor to leave the room while you have a discussion. You could say something like: 'Do you mind if we have a chat between us for a few minutes so that we can make a decision about what you have told us?' During that time, remind her that nothing can be done to her without her consent and that she should only agree to a procedure or intervention if she fully understands what she is agreeing to and feels happy with the decision.

IMPORTANT TO KNOW   *Even if at any point you feel upset or irritated by a midwife or doctor, it is a good idea to try to remain polite, as once a relationship with a health professional has broken down, communication often becomes harder.*

Vaginal Examinations

A vaginal examination (VE), is an extremely intimate procedure performed by midwives and doctors. Two fingers are lubricated and inserted into the vagina to find and assess the woman's cervix (neck of the womb) which may help to identify her progress in labour. It can feel very invasive and lead to extreme discomfort whilst the examination is being performed. Once a 'diagnosis' has been made, a woman may go through a range of emotions depending on the result, which could potentially set her labour back by diminishing her oxytocin. For a woman who has suffered any form of physical or sexual abuse, it can be a huge trigger. As her birth partner, it is very important to know that vaginal examinations are optional, and the woman can decline them at any point in her labour. Many women don't know this, or struggle to assert themselves in labour for fear of being difficult or unhelpful. I encourage all my clients to use the phrase 'not right now' when declining a VE. The midwife can document that the woman is saying no to the routine use of VEs, but leave it open so that at any point during labour, she can request one if she is ready and she feels the information will be useful.

What Does a Vaginal Examination Look For?

There are five key points that the midwife is checking when she performs a vaginal exam:

- How dilated is the cervix?
- Is it soft and thin?
- Is it short or long?
- Is it forwards or backwards?
- What position is the baby in?

> A vaginal examination cannot predict how long labour will last

What Are the Risks?

VEs are not a reliable way to measure progress, so they cannot give anyone an indication as to how long the labour will last. The result can vary depending on the person performing the exam and how relaxed the woman is at the time. Hospital guidelines say to 'offer' the woman a VE upon admission and every four hours thereafter. Many women are unaware that consenting to a VE starts a clock ticking, which exposes her to time limits. From that point onwards the midwife will want to see dilation at a rate of approximately two cm every four hours. This has the potential to dishearten the woman if she is not progressing as fast as she or her care providers would like, which in turn dramatically reduces her oxytocin. This opens up the possibility for intervention and a change from Plan A to Plan B. Vaginal examinations also come with an increased risk of the woman developing an infection. For all women, the more VEs that are performed, the greater the risk will be. The risk is significantly higher in women whose waters have broken; therefore, it is strongly recommended that a VE is avoided in this instance.

Sphincter Law

In the book *Ina May's Guide to Childbirth*, midwife Ina May Gaskin talks about 'sphincter law'. She explains that some women may have progressed to a certain stage in labour, and when a VE takes place, the cervix shrinks back away from the fingers, because it doesn't like to be poked and prodded. Midwife and author Sara Wickham calls this same phenomenon 'cervical recoil.' A common story at my pregnancy yoga class involves a woman and her birth partner leaving for hospital, believing the labour to be advanced. During a vaginal examination she is found to be 3–4 cm dilated, and whilst a little disappointed, she is advanced enough to remain in hospital and not be sent home. Within an hour or two, the woman shows signs that she is feeling an urge to push and no one believes her. In this instance, I suspect that she was more likely to have been 6 or 7 cm dilated upon arrival at the hospital, and her cervix simply closed down when the examination was performed—returning back to where it had been shortly afterwards.

Saying Yes, Please

The vast majority of women will happily accept or even request a vaginal examination because they feel that the information given during the procedure is something they want to know. Women often tell me that they like to find out if they are progressing and dilating, which is a perfectly good reason to have a VE, as the request is coming from the woman herself. She is actively consenting to the examination, which can help her feel in control.

Saying No, Thank You

If a woman is clear about not wanting to have a VE routinely, or is unsure at any point that she is offered, then her midwife should simply document this in her notes, and not pressure her into accepting. There is nothing that she has to agree to during pregnancy or labour, even if she is going against medical advice. Unfortunately, in my experience, if a medical professional wants a woman to consent to a procedure, they will persevere and try to wear her down. If she needs to be assertive, as 'No, thank you' is not working, you as the birth partner may need to ask the doctor or midwife to step outside the room. In this instance, you can calmly explain that 'no means no' and if she changes her mind, you will be the first to speak up. Rarely, you may need to ask for their names and request a change of caregiver. You can do this by speaking to the matron on shift at the time who is in charge.

Mary Cronk, a wonderful midwife who worked in the UK over many decades both as an NHS and Independent Midwife, shared a few phrases that she found helped women to assert themselves in difficult situations:

- 'Thank you so much for your advice. We will think about it very carefully and let you know our decision.'
- 'Would you like to re-consider what you have just said?'
- I'm afraid I will have to regard any further discussion as harassment.'
- 'Stop that at once!'

Other Ways to Assess Progress

As a doula, I have never performed a vaginal examination on any woman, and yet I can definitely tell when one of my clients is in labour or not. I also have a rough idea about how well she is progressing simply by noticing her behaviour. There are many clues to look for, but if in doubt, I simply sit on my hands and observe.

Here are some questions to ask yourself when trying to determine signs of active labour.

- Are her surges getting longer? They should start to creep towards about one minute in length and must be consistent. If she is having short ones and long ones with no pattern, this usually means she is still in the earlier stages.

- Is she starting to go inwards? You should notice her behaviour increasingly change, and if oxytocin is flowing, she may be very insular.

- Can you see any rhythmic behaviour? American midwife and doula Penny Simpkin calls this the three Rs: Relaxation, Rhythm and Ritual. The pregnant woman's behaviour may start to become repetitive, which helps her through each surge. I notice things like swaying or rocking of the hips, certain hand motions like squeezing and opening, moaning sounds or counting. Once she has found a movement she likes, she will use it over and over again.

- Are her feet and lower legs becoming colder? As the blood flows towards her uterus, her lower legs will become cold.

- Is she able to talk through the contractions? I never normally recommend talking to a woman during a contraction. However, if you are in a situation where, (for example) you are wondering if it might be time to call the midwife or leave to go to the hospital and you have doubts about whether she is in established labour, one trick is to ask her a question in the middle of a contraction and see if she can answer you. If she has to wait until the contraction has gone, and needs a bit of recovery time afterwards before sleepily asking you to repeat what you just said, she is more than likely to be in established labour and it is a good time to call.

PAULA'S STORY Paula was in strong labour when she arrived at the hospital several hours after labour began with her first child. As she walked from the door to the desk in the triage area, she had two contractions, one more whilst she stood at the desk, and another two on the way down the corridor and into the assessment room. She struggled to get onto the bed where the midwife had invited her to 'hop on so I can check to see if you are in labour'. She had been in the company of the midwife for less than 10 minutes. Her partner, who knew Paula wanted to avoid all vaginal examinations, explained this to the midwife and asked if the pool room was available that day. The midwife, following hospital guidelines, encouraged the VE and tried to persuade Paula to have the procedure by explaining that she would not be able to enter the labour ward and give her the pool room unless established labour was determined. During this time, she'd had several long and powerful contractions, and her partner looked at the midwife in despair. He then, using a calm voice, invited the midwife to kindly sit and observe Paula for the next 10 minutes without speaking or moving. He said that if at that point, she still felt that Paula was not in established labour, then they could have another discussion. The midwife, looking quite embarrassed, scuttled off and began to prepare the pool room for her.

. . . .

Going Too Far

Unfortunately on a couple of occasions I have witnessed a vaginal examination being taken too far.

On one occasion my client had consented to the exam; however, whilst the midwife's hand was inside her, she performed a stretch and sweep of the woman's membranes without permission. This was something the midwife decided to do to my client without any discussion, and my client was furious. She had been in extreme discomfort during the examination, and the midwife had 'shushed' at her, implying she was being ridiculous. Had it been explained to my client in advance that a stretch and sweep of the cervix was an option, she would have been able to ask questions about what was involved, and decide if she wanted to give her consent or not.

The midwife apologised at my client's discomfort as she removed her hand, but gave the 'good news' that she had given her a really good stretch and that things should tick along nicely now. My client felt violated.

A woman who is consenting to a vaginal examination should not have to specify that she would like to have a discussion before an extra procedure is carried out.

I explain to all my clients and their birth partners that they should ask a few questions before consenting to any intervention, including what is involved, and whether there are likely to be any other actions set in motion because of the decision. She can ask:

- What will you be looking for when you are performing the examination?
- Do you agree to tell me exactly what you are doing at all times and ask my permission first if you would like to carry out any other procedures?
- Do you agree to stop immediately if I ask you to?

She does not have to be touched by anyone who has not specifically explained what they are about to do. I encourage her to find her voice in every moment that doesn't feel right, as it is much easier to ask a medical professional to stop and remove their hands, than to spend the rest of her life re-living that experience through flashbacks.

Postnatal VEs

At some stage within an hour or two of the baby being born, the woman will be offered an examination to check for vaginal and rectal tearing. This involves placing two fingers inside the vagina to check for grazes or tears, and a finger inside the anus to check for any additional tearing in the back passage. The tears are measured in the degree of damage to the perineum (the area between the vaginal opening and the rectum) from first to fourth degree. As you can imagine, this can be another very invasive procedure for some women, especially if they have declined routine vaginal examinations throughout labour for a reason that is important to them. The expectation that she 'has' to have this additional check can come as a shock. These examinations can also be declined, and not all tears have to be sutured (sewn together). Usually a graze and a first degree tear are left to heal naturally. A second degree tear may be left alone, or it may be recommended to be sutured, depending on where the tear is and the woman's preference. Many of my clients have declined being sutured, as the body heals quickly within a short space of time with less risk of infection, just like any cut or graze to the skin. In comparison, a third and fourth degree tear will need to be sutured in theatre, as these involve many layers of tissue, possibly including repair to internal and external sphincters.

Speak to the woman during the antenatal period and discuss her thoughts around these procedures, and do your research into what tearing involves, so that if necessary you can ask questions on the day about her options. If she has any concerns, she will be able to raise them in advance with her midwife or doctor and discuss the pros and cons.

Post-Birth Discussions

The women I know who feel listened to and in control of the decision-making process throughout their pregnancy, labour and birth, almost always come out the other side feeling extremely positive about their experience, no matter what twists and turns it may take on the day. In the 20 years I have been involved in supporting thousands of women and their partners during this process, either in person or via a class or course, I have learned that the psychological effect of the birth experience can fade, but never goes away. A woman will remember her birth stories for the rest of her life, and whilst a healthy baby is important, it is definitely not all that matters. During the postnatal period she is especially vulnerable, and one wrong word or action can leave her feeling a range of emotions, including failure or guilt if the birth did not go well. In this instance, she needs to recognise that how she feels about her birth experience is completely separate from how she feels about her baby.

My recommendation to you as her birth partner is to take time to have some dedicated discussions about the birth in the postnatal period. Try to schedule a session within the first two weeks after the birth. If you think it necessary, you could have another conversation about how she is feeling at some stage in the months that follow, as it might be interesting to see if her thoughts about the birth have changed. Often a woman will gloss over her true feelings in the early postnatal days, and may be able to express herself more clearly once a period of time has passed. If you are her spouse, then make sure you tell her that you want to schedule time to talk specifically about the birth. Watch her closely as she describes the experience and the way she feels about it, particularly if it was not what she had expected. It is a good idea to fill in the gaps if there are details she has forgotten, but recognise that her version of events is always the one that you should validate. You can, of course, also talk freely about your own feelings, and share with her what you went through. Sometimes, a birth partner can struggle with feelings of failure and guilt. These are important to vocalise, particularly if you are feeling this way yourself. During the session make sure that you:

- Let her talk about her experience freely.
- Acknowledge her feelings.
- Praise her decisions.
- Do not diminish what she went through.
- Take ownership of your own thoughts and feelings about the birth.

If you think the woman would benefit from a professional review of the birth, then you could recommend she access the birth listening service at her local hospital, where a dedicated midwife will facilitate a meeting for you both to attend. At that meeting, the midwife will be able to talk through the notes that were written during her labour, fill in gaps and answer any questions that either of you may have. If she prefers, she can request that a copy of those notes be sent to her. If she reads them and sees words or comments that she doesn't understand, she can call the hospital for an explanation. It is worth knowing, however, that it can feel very upsetting for some women to read information that was documented in their birth notes that they might not like or agree with. For this reason, it is best that she read them with someone else present. I have heard of women who read comments that indicate she 'gave consent' when she didn't, or 'requested' (a procedure) when she didn't. I have also heard about other negative comments like 'failure to progress' in the first stage, or 'poor maternal effort' during the second stage (meaning she wasn't pushing effectively). These comments can be hurtful, so if she doesn't want to speak to an NHS midwife, she can book a birth exploration session privately with a doula or independent midwife who offers this service. It can be very healing for a woman to talk to an experienced professional and can help answer some of the questions she may have going around in her head. In some instances, I would also recommend asking if she would be prepared to write down her experience and either keep it for herself or potentially offer it as feedback to the local hospital in the area where she gave birth. Some women may decide to make a formal complaint if the circumstances warrant it. It is a very personal choice, which some women will decide to pursue and others will not. If she wants to look into giving feedback, she can contact her local MVP (Maternity Voices Partnership) representative in England, or Maternity Services Liaison Committee (MSLC) in Scotland, Ireland and Wales, who will be able to deliver the feedback on her behalf. She can also contact PALS (Patient Advocate Liaison Services) at the hospital she was booked under.

Birth Trauma and Post-Traumatic Stress Disorder

Post-traumatic stress disorder (PTSD) is starting to become more widely recognised throughout the birth industry. It is my hope that health professionals will look more closely at the way they speak to women during birth, because trauma can be lessened when the woman is treated with kindness and respect. Experiencing trauma can often leave the woman and/or her birth partner with feelings they may not want to acknowledge, with some preferring to avoid talking about their birth altogether. Many don't realise they have experienced a trauma, and some leave it buried deep down until they are pregnant with a subsequent child. It can hit them like a tonne of bricks when they remember that they have to go through birth again, especially if it was well and truly parked at the back of their mind until that point. When it does come to the surface, it is highly likely to shape the decisions that the woman makes about her future birth, often including hiring additional support (a doula or independent midwife), and having a deep determination to avoid the same scenarios. This is why I often see high-risk women giving birth at home, or low-risk women having a planned c-section. These women need time and extra support to explore their options and their emotions over the course of the pregnancy when deciding on their own personal Plan A.

QUICK RECAP

Here are the main things to remember when realising that a healthy baby is not all that matters.

- **Instincts.** Remember that no one knows the woman like the woman knows herself. She should trust her instincts and take ownership of the decisions made about her care where possible.
- **T-BRAIN.** Become familiar with the T-BRAIN tool and question everything. This applies even if she already knows she is going to agree to any recommendations given to her.
- **No means no!** If she says no, raises a hand to say no, or shakes her head in the middle of a contraction, she is clearly stating No! She can always use the response 'not right now', to be clear that she is not refusing, but politely declining in that moment whatever is being offered.

- **Vaginal examinations.** Talk about her feelings around vaginal examinations. Make sure she understands that she can accept or decline. You should also discuss her feelings about a post-birth examination.
- **Post-birth discussion.** Schedule a post-birth discussion session to talk about how the birth was for her, and also to give you the opportunity to share anything from your perspective.

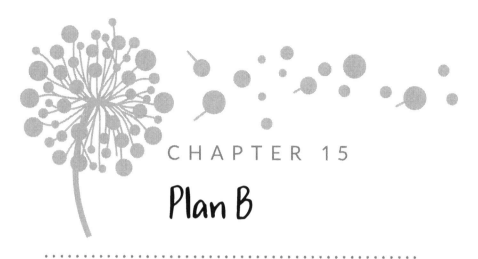

CHAPTER 15

Plan B

. . . .

You don't always need a plan. Sometimes you just need to breathe, trust, let go and see what happens.

–Mandy Hale

For some women, as pregnancy progresses, it can become apparent that the dream birth they have been planning may no longer be possible. A health concern can develop for either the woman or the baby, or another unforeseen reason can arise—including the possibility that the woman herself simply decides on a new plan. If this occurs during pregnancy, then it should at least allow for some preparation time and the opportunity to discuss new ideas about birth options with her care providers. As always, it is important that she questions everything, because in an era where fear of litigation hangs over everyone, a doctor or midwife may practice defensively. What I mean is that in some cases, a woman can be encouraged to accept an intervention when it might not actually be relevant to her personal situation—she just happened to tick a box. She may be automatically switched from the low-risk pathway to a high-risk one, with the reasons not always being clear to her. In this chapter, I have listed some of the more common scenarios I have come across, to give you an idea of any issues that might occur with the woman you are supporting. It is not essential that you read all the sections of this chapter, but it is important that you don't skip it altogether in case a medical issue arises during labour, and a switch to Plan B becomes necessary.

IMPORTANT TO KNOW *If a woman needs to ask questions about her options and any recommendations that have been given, remind her that she can also ask for evidence or research to back up any claims made by the doctor or midwife. If she chooses to decline a recommendation, she does not need to justify that decision.*

> It is not a woman's job to explain
> why she doesn't want to consent!

Plan B in Pregnancy:
When Her Plans Go out the Window

At some stage during the pregnancy, she might:

- Discover that the baby has a medical condition that requires it to be born early.
- Develop a condition that may require more serious monitoring.
- Discover that her baby is not following the growth chart, and be called in for extra scans.
- Learn that the baby's position or placenta position make it impossible to give birth vaginally.
- Change her mind based on her own personal circumstances, which may or may not be out of her control.

Due to any of the reasons above, the woman may reach a point in the pregnancy where an induction or c-section is recommended, or an alternative to her original plan is suggested. Whatever the reason, changing her plans will most likely feel very disappointing, and this should be validated.

Even in the event that any decision appears to be 'out of her hands', and the reasons are obviously serious, the woman should still always have the final say. Use the T-BRAIN tool in Chapter 14 to ask questions about her own personal circumstances to ensure she fully understands what she is consenting to.

Baby Measuring Small

Towards the end of the second trimester, during midwife or hospital appointments, women are assessed to check for growth of the baby. The midwife will plot the growth on a chart to record progress. Sometimes this indicates that the growth of the baby has slowed or stopped. If the midwife is concerned, the woman may be offered an extra ultrasound scan to look specifically at the baby's growth. This situation is often called small for gestational age (SGA), small for dates (SFD), or Intrauterine Growth Restriction (IUGR). Most babies that are smaller than expected will be healthy, but up to 10% of pregnancies will be affected by IUGR and will need close monitoring during the remainder of the pregnancy. In some cases the baby will need to be born earlier than expected. In this instance, the mother will be offered steroids to mature her baby's lungs in preparation for a premature birth, and depending on the gestation and health of the baby, a discussion about induction versus c-section will need to take place. At this stage, you can also enquire about paediatric support and what is involved in the care of the baby during the early postnatal period in the event that he or she may require it. The hospital may offer a visit to the SCBU if the doctors know that your baby is going to have to spend some time there.

IMPORTANT TO KNOW *Growth scans are notoriously inaccurate, and there is a 15% margin of error on either side of the measurement you are given. If the woman has had one scan that shows a smaller weight baby, but then the next scan does not, she should ask about being referred back to low-risk care if no other factors are involved.*

Baby Measuring Big

Conversely, the baby could be suspected as measuring bigger than average. In this instance, in addition to a growth scan, the woman may also be offered a glucose tolerance test (GTT) for Gestational Diabetes, leading to a high-risk diagnosis. The average weight of a newborn baby is around 3.4 kg (7 lb 8 oz), with a baby considered to be larger than normal weighing 4kg (8lb 13oz) or more. Macrosomia (the medical term, which literally means "big body") will apply to approximately 1 in 10 babies, and of those, most will have absolutely no problem being born vaginally. Dr Rachel Reed in her blog **midwifethinking.com** says: 'The only way to accurately assess the weight of a baby is to weigh it after birth. Clinical assessment, i.e. palpating and measuring pregnant bumps, is incorrect more than 50% of the time (Chauhan et al. 2005). Even the best available method—measuring the baby's abdomen with an ultrasound—only predicts the weight of the baby within 15% of their actual weight (Rossi et al. 2013)'. So whilst it is important for the woman to be made aware that her baby may be measuring larger than average, it is also important to recognise that the negative effects of additional scans, discussions about shoulder dystocia, and offers of an early induction, can leave damaging seeds of doubt in the woman's mind that she is capable of giving birth safely. The label 'big baby' can become a self-fulfilling prophecy, with the woman's own subconscious mind imagining growing a baby to huge proportions. This can lead to her having to endure a more painful labour, thinking that not only could the baby get stuck, but her own body could be damaged in the process. In most cases the new 'high-risk' label means the woman may be denied options around place of birth, and is told that she is no longer 'allowed' to give birth at home or in an MLU. The recommendation of induction, even though there is no reason to suspect that she will have any issue giving birth whatsoever, pretty much guarantees that she will be unable to labour in an upright, gravity-assisted position. For this reason, induction is listed as a risk factor for shoulder dystocia, because of the pelvic outlet restrictions resulting from women giving birth on their backs. The irony of this recommendation is not lost on me!

IMPORTANT TO KNOW   *As mentioned before, growth scans are often inaccurate, and the woman will need a lot of reassurance from you if it is even suggested that her baby is bigger than average. If an induction is recommended, use the T-BRAIN tool in Chapter 14 to weigh up the benefits and risks of either accepting the induction or declining. There are plenty of really useful websites and blogs that cover this subject in detail, such as* **sarawickham.com,** **midwifethinking.com** *by Dr Rachel Reed, and* **evidencebasedbirth.com** *by Rebecca Dekker.*

Placenta Previa

Placenta previa (or low-lying placenta) occurs when the placenta is partially or totally covering the mother's cervix, effectively 'blocking the exit route'. In 90% of cases, as the baby develops, the uterus grows and the placenta will move upwards and out of the way, no longer a concern. A low-lying placenta can cause bleeding throughout pregnancy, which can be alarming for the woman but doesn't usually cause a problem to the pregnancy. The hardest part is that the woman can be left waiting a long time to find out about her options for birth, as there is a small possibility the placenta will remain low, and the baby will have to be born via c-section. Most women will be offered a scan at 32 weeks, with a small minority waiting until 36 weeks for a definite answer.

Twins or Multiples

Discovering that there is more than one baby on board immediately puts a woman on the high-risk pathway, and she will be advised to have regular scans. This is because of the level of potential complications that a multiple pregnancy can bring. There are amazing resources out there for parents-to-be of twins and multiples, including Twins Trust (**twinstrust. org**), so it should be easy to find information if you are supporting a woman through a multiple pregnancy. Hospitals have their guidelines, but it is still the woman's choice to decide how she wants to proceed throughout her pregnancy and birth. If she would prefer to opt for a vaginal birth, most hospitals require the first (lowest) baby to be head down, and the babies to be similar in size. For any other variation, you can still expect a personalised care plan. You should not assume that she has to have a c-section if she doesn't want one.

Transverse Lie

Regardless of what position a baby is in throughout the pregnancy, towards the end, most babies will turn so that their head is down. Rarely, (approximately 1 in 300) a baby will lie in a sideways position across the belly, called a transverse lie. Depending on the circumstances of each individual woman, she may be offered the opportunity for an experienced doctor to turn the baby using a manual procedure where they physically try to manoeuvre the baby round using their hands. This is called an external cephalic version (ECV). If she chooses to accept, this will be done in hospital and the baby monitored carefully, as there are risks associated with ECV. These risks include rupture of membranes (waters around the baby), and heavy bleeding. If an ECV is declined, or not successful, a c-section will become necessary.

Breech

A baby whose head is up under its mother's ribcage is called a breech baby. Most will be head down by about 36–37 weeks, but approximately 3% of babies will remain in a persistent breech position.

There are three main types of breech:

1. Frank breech—the baby's legs are straight up in front of its body in a V shape, so its feet are up near its face.

2. Complete breech—the baby is in a sitting position with its legs crossed in front of its body and its feet near its bottom.

3. Footling breech—one or both of the baby's feet are hanging below its bottom, so the foot or feet are in position to be born first.

If a baby remains in the breech position beyond 36 weeks, similar to a baby in the transverse position, the woman may be offered an ECV. If the baby successfully turns, she will be left to continue her pregnancy. If not, then she is most likely to be offered a c-section. If the woman you are supporting would prefer to give birth vaginally, then it is worth speaking to the hospitals locally to see how many vaginal breech births were achieved in the previous 12 months. This will help her to identify which ones have the most experience, and will give her confidence in the location she chooses.

IMPORTANT TO KNOW *There are some natural ways to encourage a breech baby to turn. Have a look at* **spinningbabies.com** *for ideas on positions to adopt during pregnancy that may help. Another idea is to visit an acupuncturist who can use a technique called moxibustion. This is a traditional Chinese medicine used to heat specific energy points on the woman's feet.*

Gestational Diabetes

In some cases a woman may be invited for a glucose tolerance test (GTT), because of one of the following: her midwife finds high blood sugar levels in her urine during a routine appointment, she has a high BMI, she has a family history of diabetes, or the midwife has concerns that the baby is measuring bigger than expected. This test is optional, and the woman can do her own research regarding its accuracy before she decides to accept or decline. If gestational diabetes is diagnosed, an induction of labour may be recommended for several reasons, including concerns that the baby will grow too big. Again, this is a recommendation and is still something she can discuss and potentially delay or decline based on her own personal circumstances.

Pre-eclampsia

This is a disorder that is detected through urine and blood pressure checks performed routinely at each midwife appointment. Most women are typically unaware that they have pre-eclampsia before they are diagnosed; however, some will describe feeling unwell and may have begun to develop symptoms that can include fluid retention in the face, hands and feet (oedema), severe headache, blurred vision and pain just below the ribs. Although many cases are typically mild, the condition, which affects black women 60% more than white women, is important to know about, as it can lead to serious complications for both mother and baby if it's not monitored and treated. The only way to cure pre-eclampsia is to give birth to the baby, so in many cases it may become necessary for the baby to be born prematurely.

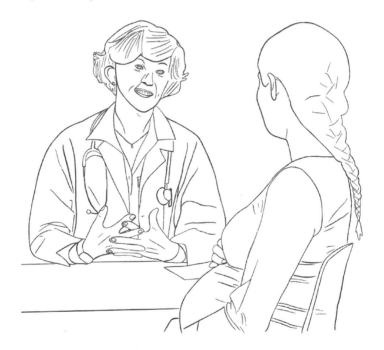

Group B Strep

Group B strep (GBS) is a bacteria that lives harmlessly in the vagina, and can very rarely (1 in 1,750 pregnancies) transfer to the baby, leading it to develop a serious infection after birth. There is no NHS routine screening programme for GBS, but women can opt for a private test. If a woman is found to be GBS-positive at the time she is tested, it does not mean she will still have GBS present in the vagina when her labour begins, as it is common for the bacteria to come and go. She will, however, as a matter of routine, be offered the use of IV antibiotics in labour. If she accepts, she will be asked to arrive at the hospital during early labour to be given antibiotics through a cannula in her hand every four hours until the baby arrives. Each dose takes approximately 20 minutes to administer, so mobility can be limited. Babies are at higher risk of developing GBS if:

- They are premature (born before 37 weeks).
- The mother's waters broke over a prolonged period of time (36 hours or more).
- The mother has had multiple vaginal examinations.
- The mother develops an elevated temperature during labour— a sign of infection.

In any of these instances, with no prior testing, the woman will be offered antibiotics as a preventative measure. As there are negative side effects to the use of antibiotics, which will affect both the woman and the baby, she should do a lot of research before making a decision to accept or decline.

IMPORTANT TO KNOW *Women are not routinely screened for GBS; however, women who are planning a home birth or want to give birth in an MLU may be tested for this without realising or consenting. Please make sure that you remind the woman you are supporting that she has the right to ask any care provider taking blood tests, urine samples or swab tests, what exactly they will be testing for, and how that will impact her choices for birth. That way she has the ability to accept or decline.*

Obstetric Cholestasis

Obstetric cholestasis (OC) is a disorder that affects a pregnant woman's liver. It is caused by a build up of bile acids and other substances which then leak into the woman's bloodstream. The most obvious way to spot OC is that the mother develops extreme itching, particularly on the hands and feet, although it can be all over the body and can be worse at night. Whilst itching is common in pregnancy, affecting around 23% of women, only a small proportion (0.7%) will actually have OC. For women with the disorder, there is a higher risk of premature birth and stillbirth, so once diagnosed, a woman is usually monitored closely with the option of an induction if their bile acid levels rise.

Premature Birth

Sometimes, babies are born early (defined as anytime before 37 weeks), and it can be a huge shock and a very scary experience for both parents. In the event that it becomes obvious the woman you are supporting is going into labour prematurely, contact the hospital immediately. In most cases, she will be given steroid injections to mature the baby's lungs and in some cases she may be given drugs to try and slow or stop the labour. If labour is inevitable, don't forget to check her list of preferences written on the birth plan, as there may still be some that apply to her. If you have time, show them to the midwife and discuss ways to help achieve as many as possible. Once the baby is born, they may need to be taken to the special care baby unit (SCBU). The staff there will make every effort for the mother to have skin to skin with the baby as soon as possible.

IMPORTANT TO KNOW Premature babies really benefit from optimal cord clamping, so if a paediatrician is called to attend, ask them if they are happy to do checks on the baby close to the mother so that the cord can be left to stop pulsating. If the woman is keen to breast feed, she can express colostrum/ milk and this will be given to the baby either by tube or bottle until breastfeeding can be initiated.

Reduced Fetal Movements

Fetal movements are usually felt for the first time around 20 weeks of pregnancy. It can be later for women whose placenta is situated at the front, and much earlier for some women, particularly those who have been pregnant before. Kicks Count (**kickscount.org.uk**), an organisation set up to educate parents about fetal movement, says: 'There is no set number of normal movements. Your baby will have their own pattern of movements that you should get to know. From 16–24 weeks onwards you should feel the baby move more and more up until 32 weeks then stay roughly the same until you give birth'. Their overall recommendation is that the woman gets to know what is normal for her baby, and she can then keep track of its movements to know that it's maintaining a regular pattern. If reduced fetal movements (RFM) are suspected, encourage her to be checked out by her midwife or at the hospital. The RCOG Green-top guidelines for RFM say: 'Women should be reassured that 70% of pregnancies with a single episode of RFM are uncomplicated. If after discussion with the clinician it is clear that the woman does not have RFM, in the absence of further risk factors and the presence of a normal fetal heart rate on auscultation (listening to the baby's heart rate), there should be no need to follow up with further investigations. If there is a concern with the baby, then conversations should take place regarding how to continue to monitor the baby until the point where labour begins or a c-section becomes necessary. If an induction is offered, it is worth talking in detail about the effects that it may have on the baby before making a decision. If there is already an indication that the baby isn't coping in the womb, you can seriously question whether it's a good choice to put it under more stress during the induction. In which case, you can ask about going straight to the option of a c-section. With your support, the woman should ask as many questions as she can, in order to make a well informed decision about the personal circumstances that she is facing.

IMPORTANT TO KNOW   *If the woman you are supporting attends two or more appointments for RFM then she is immediately determined to be high risk, and her birth options seriously diminish. She will still have access to all the facilities that labour wards have to offer, and could still decide to give birth at home if she wanted to, but she is likely to be outside of the criteria for most MLUs. In this instance, you will need to speak to her about Plan B.*

Induction of Labour

An induction of labour is the process in which a woman goes into the hospital to begin interventions that will encourage her cervix to soften, ripen and dilate in order for her baby to be born. It can be offered to a woman because it has been decided that it is not safe for her pregnancy to continue, or it could be that she has passed her due date and the guidelines of the hospital she is booked under state that she should be induced because she has no signs of labour. To put it bluntly, she simply ran out of time. Midwife and author Dr Sara Wickham has written a book and many useful articles about induction that you can read on her website, **sarawickham. com**. Here she states many times that induction isn't compulsory: "It's not law!" She points out that in most cases, induction is not what women want. They would prefer not to accept it but were given a date as if they didn't have a choice in the matter. In her book *Inducing Labour,* she says, 'It is important to mention that induction of labour (which predicts roughly when women will give birth) may occasionally also be more convenient for the hospital, midwife or doctor. Sometimes women request induction themselves. Women can face a lot of pressure from all sorts of people towards the end of pregnancy ("Haven't you had it yet?!"). Perhaps this is because our modern culture values efficiency, productivity and punctuality, and being overdue in any context is seen as a negative thing. But women have the right to make their own decision about this and any other intervention they are offered, and guidelines are just that: a guide.' Sara describes herself as a midwife who believes that it is generally better not to intervene unless it is really warranted.

Many of the women I speak to have heard stories about how awful induction can be, and it is obvious to them without reading a single research paper that there is a greater chance of intervention and c-section. There are, of course, plenty of positive stories about induction, but there is no getting away from the fact that it is an incredibly overused procedure that in many cases can be avoided. I think if the woman you are supporting has researched and decided that she is happy to accept an induction of labour, then there are many ways to make it a positive experience. Suggestions include downloading movies, buying lovely books and settling in for the time it takes, with a smile. It is an opportunity to do nothing until labour starts. When she does begin to feel contractions, refer to the other chapters in this book about positions and skills like hypnobirthing, which can be very effective during any labour. If, however, the woman you are supporting is keen to avoid an induction, then look around locally to see what the options are, as different hospitals offer induction at different dates in the pregnancy. She can, of course, decline an induction and wait for labour to start in its own time. This is common if a woman believes her EDD was wrong, and at her 12-week scan she was given a date that was different from her own. A small proportion of women give birth between 42 and 44 weeks, and during that time, most will attend the hospital for regular checks and scans to ensure that the baby is doing well as they wait it out.

Bishop's Score

If an induction is recommended, the woman will be offered a vaginal examination, during which the midwife will assess the cervix to check for signs of: dilation, position, length and softness. Known as a 'Bishop's score', this assessment is used to try to identify if the woman will go into labour soon, and if the induction is likely to work. A score higher than 9 indicates that labour will probably start without the need for induction. A score that is lower than 5 suggests that labour would not begin without induction. A score lower than 3 means that induction will probably take a long time or may not work at all. In this instance, she must plan for the long haul. You should prepare yourself for the fact that it might well take many days for labour to begin.

IMPORTANT TO KNOW *The woman can ask for her Bishop's score, as it is not always shared as a matter of routine. This may help her if she is trying to decide between accepting or declining an induction.*

Methods of Induction

Cervical sweep

A 'sweep' is an attempt to stimulate a woman's cervix into action, so that labour begins. The procedure, which is usually performed by a midwife, involves them placing their finger inside the woman's vagina and making a sweeping movement to separate the membranes that surround the baby from the cervix. Most women are offered a sweep from around 40 weeks pregnant and beyond. If it works, the woman will start showing signs of labour within 48 hours, helping her to avoid an induction. A sweep can be very uncomfortable, and there is the potential for some bleeding afterwards.

IMPORTANT TO KNOW *A common issue with a cervical sweep is that for some women it can stimulate the cervix enough to produce contractions. However, because the baby might not be ready to be born, they eventually fizzle out, leaving the woman exhausted. In this scenario, she should rest as much as possible.*

Hormones

The hormone prostaglandin is required to soften and ripen the cervix. When an induction begins, the first step in the process, based on the results of the Bishop's Score, may be to insert a tampon-shaped pessary or gel into the vagina that contains a synthetic version of the hormone. This can take a few hours or a few days to work. The woman will be initially assessed after 6, 12 or 24 hours, depending on which brand of drug is used. In some cases, the birth partner is sent home over night while the prostaglandins take their time to work.

IMPORTANT TO KNOW *Sometimes a woman can 'overstimulate' when a prostaglandin drug is used. You might notice that the contractions come quickly with very little break in between. If this happens to the woman you are supporting* *then tell the midwife. If there is a tampon in place, she will be able to remove it which might help. If the baby is not coping, a c-section may be recommended.*

Cervical Ripening Balloon

In some hospitals, they might offer the option of using a silicone balloon that is inserted into the vagina through a catheter. The balloon is then inflated and filled with saline, which will hopefully begin to apply pressure to the walls of the cervix, causing the hormone prostaglandin to be produced. If the cervix softens and opens, the procedure has been successful, and the balloon may eventually drop out on its own or can be removed by the midwife after 24 hours. This method is drug free.

Breaking Waters

If the woman's cervix successfully softens and moves round to the front with the use of prostaglandins or the balloon, and contractions have not yet begun, it is assumed that the next stage is to break the bag of waters around the baby. The midwife must be able to get a finger into the cervix and can then use an 'amnihook' (which looks like a long crochet needle) to break the waters. This will hopefully be enough to trigger contractions on its own.

Oxytocin Drip

If a woman's cervix is already ripened and she has no contractions, or they are considered irregular or short in length, doctors can prescribe a synthetic oxytocin drug that the midwife can administer through a drip. The drug, called 'syntocinon' will be given in small doses (at first) and will then be increased slowly to stimulate contractions and dilate the cervix. This also gives the woman's endorphin levels a chance to rise at the same time.

IMPORTANT TO KNOW *This drip can be turned up or down when necessary. Sometimes the contractions produced are strong and the woman may choose to have an epidural if she finds the intensity too much too soon.*

During an Induction

The induction bay, typically on the postnatal ward, may have several women who are all at different stages of the process. Once the induction is working, and the woman is contracting well, she may still be left for long periods of time until labour becomes established. It can be difficult for the woman to be on an induction bay, as there is often little space and virtually no privacy other than a curtain around the bed. It is important to keep her in an optimal position where possible. If she wants some pain relief, and you think she is ready to be moved to labour ward, you will need to speak to the midwives on her behalf.

. . . .

TEGAN'S STORY During pregnancy, Tegan was told by several of her friends that there is a perception that black women have a higher pain threshold and that she should 'exaggerate pain felt during contractions' in order to be taken seriously. She told me: 'This in my mind was contradictory to all we'd learnt on our antenatal course, and I chose not to do this. However, reflecting on my experience, during my induction, I really did have to insist on being examined on the ward because my contractions were so regular and so intense. It turns out I was 8 cm dilated and should have gone down to labour ward a lot sooner and offered suitable pain relief.'

. . . .

Unfortunately Tegan's experience highlights a common issue within the induction process. Women describe being left alone and 'forgotten' for many hours. This can be really scary, especially if the contractions are intense and the woman believes she is still in the very early stages of labour, with no idea about how she will cope with what is ahead. Many express that they were not believed when their labour was quick, leading to their receiving no support and no pain relief when required. In my opinion, this is why a large number of women who begin labour with an induction will go on to require a c-section.

Further, Tegan's experience is indicative of some of the issues that can arise more often for any woman from a culturally diverse or lower socio-economic background, who are sometimes misunderstood or sidelined by medical professionals. This has been highlighted in a recent report that shows that statistically, black women are five times more likely to die of a pregnancy-related complication than white women, and Asian women three times more likely (see the Resources section at the back of the book).

Augmentation of Labour

If labour has already started, but has slowed or stalled, the doctor may suggest using the same drug given in an induction—syntocinon—to increase the frequency, duration and intensity of contractions after the onset of spontaneous labour.

IMPORTANT TO KNOW *With a labour that has slowed or stalled, it is likely that the woman's own oxytocin production has diminished. You can go back to basics and ensure she is feeling relaxed and calm, turn out the lights, and stay quiet. You can also consider using homeopathy (caulophyllum), aromatherapy (clary sage), nipple stimulation, or change of position. More likely, all she needs is to eat, hydrate, and rest for a while and the contractions will come back on their own.*

Cascade of Interventions

Once one intervention has taken place, it is often the case that more will follow. It is important to be prepared for this. If you are able to recognise what is coming, you as the birth partner can be prepared to support her in a much more empowering way. It is still important for her to produce as much oxytocin as possible, so ideally discussions should always be kept to a minimum. However, I would definitely recommend you bring her out of her 'bubble' if you think she can benefit from hearing some vital information about a future possible procedure that will give her overall control. This will make it easier for her to overcome any twists and turns her birth may take. The most difficult experience to bounce back from is when the reason to switch to Plan B was not maternal choice, and a cascade of interventions then followed.

I typically see more intervention used when:

- She arrives at the hospital or calls the midwife to her home birth too early.
- She doesn't eat or drink enough to sustain the contractions or her energy.
- Gas and air use begins early (around 4 cm).
- A second VE determines no progress since the last VE, indicating a plateau.
- Labour slows down and syntocinon is given to speed up contractions.
- She labour's overnight with slow progress and is unable to rest and 'flop' to conserve her energy.
- She has an epidural.
- She begins pushing without an overwhelming urge, leading to an assisted birth.

IMPORTANT TO KNOW   *If intervention occurs as a direct result of a decision she makes, then you should confidently praise her afterwards and share with her that you would have done exactly the same in her situation. A positive experience is always possible if she is consulted at each step and makes her own decisions.*

Home Birth to Hospital Birth

For some women, switching from Plan A to Plan B means giving up a dream to give birth at home. Assuming the woman is already in established labour and has been contracting for some time, she may transfer into hospital for the following reasons.

- Progress may be slow, and she becomes exhausted.
- The baby may not be coping well, and it's heart rate is showing signs of concern.
- The woman may prefer to transfer for pain relief.

- The woman may instinctively feel like something is wrong.
- The baby may pass significant meconium (baby's first poo), which can be a sign of distress.
- The woman may be asked to go to the hospital because at the time you call for a midwife to attend, there is no one available. (In this instance, you can still stay at home and insist that they find a midwife to assist you).

Postnatal Transfer

If a transfer becomes necessary after the birth, it may be because there are concerns for mother or baby. The reasons may include heavy bleeding, baby having breathing difficulties, mum or baby showing signs of an infection, or a retained placenta. The paramedics will be called and will always do their best to keep mum and baby together, unless the baby needs immediate care. In my experience, it is unlikely that the ambulance crew will let the birth partner travel in the ambulance, as they would usually have a midwife sit with the woman in the back and there is simply not enough room. In this instance, you would follow behind with the bags, meeting the woman at the hospital. If the baby is well, you may even be expected to take the baby in the car with you. I recommend that every labouring woman have a birth bag containing all she might need for her birth, which can be picked up and taken wherever she goes.

IMPORTANT TO KNOW   *Not all transfers will require an ambulance, and many women can decline and be driven to the hospital by their partners, depending on the circumstances. Practice putting the baby's car seat in and out of the car ahead of time so that it is familiar to you.*

MLU to Hospital Birth

For the same reasons listed in the home birth section, a woman who is giving birth in a midwife-led, birth centre-type setting may need to switch to consultant-led care. If this happens during labour, it will require the woman to be transported to the main labour ward. If she is in an alongside MLU attached to a hospital, then the transfer is reasonably straightforward. In most cases there is a door that separates the two, and the transfer takes minutes; however, other hospitals have their MLU in a different part of the building and the transfer time might take longer. Typically, the MLU will arrange an appointment with her around 36 weeks, where they will discuss transfer times. If the woman gives birth in a standalone MLU, then she will be transferred to the main hospital in an ambulance.

IMPORTANT TO KNOW *After the baby is born, assuming the birth was reasonably straightforward, many MLUs will accept the woman back for the early postnatal period, if they have space for her to return.*

Assisted Birth

If the woman is in the pushing stage for a prolonged period of time and is struggling to move her baby down, or if the baby is deemed to be in an unfavourable position, a doctor may offer to help with two methods of assistance (also known as instrumental birth). The doctor will decide between a ventouse (vacuum cup) or forceps (tongs). The decision between the two will be made after the doctor performs a vaginal examination and feels for the position of the baby's head; then a discussion with the woman should take place. If the woman is unmedicated at this point, she will be given an anaesthetic injection to numb the area, and it is most likely that they will need to widen the vaginal opening with an episiotomy (small cut). The woman will then require stitches after the baby is born to repair the cut. The **nhs.uk** website describes the following differences between the two options:

A **ventouse** (vacuum cup) is attached to the baby's head by suction. A soft or hard plastic or metal cup is attached by a tube to a suction device. The cup fits firmly on to your baby's head. During a contraction and with the help of your pushing, the obstetrician or midwife gently pulls to help deliver your baby.

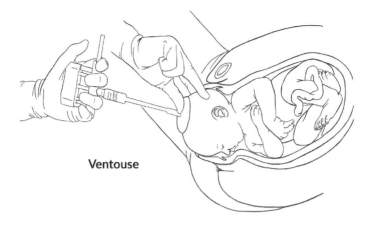

Ventouse

Forceps are smooth metal instruments that look like large spoons or tongs. They're curved to fit around the baby's head. The forceps are carefully positioned around your baby's head and joined together at the handles. With a contraction and your pushing, an obstetrician gently pulls to help deliver your baby. There are different types of forceps. Some are specifically designed to turn the baby to the correct position to be born, such as if your baby is lying facing upwards (occipito-posterior position) or to one side (occipito-lateral position).

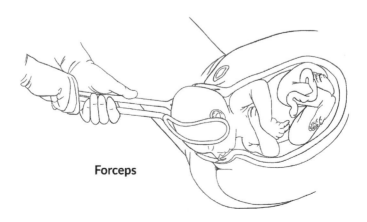

Forceps

According to RCOG, approximately one in eight women have an assisted vaginal birth, and this is more likely (one in three) for women having their first baby. These statistics are, in my opinion, shockingly high, and whether this many are actually necessary is definitely debatable. You can help the woman you are supporting by understanding that there are some key factors that increase the chances of her requiring assistance during the pushing stage and avoid them where possible. She may require assistance if:

* she is unable to adopt a position that facilitates the baby moving through the pelvis easily.
* it is perceived her baby might be 'big'.
* she has had an epidural during labour.
* her baby has remained in a persistent posterior position (back to back).
* she is being guided to push and therefore not pushing with an overwhelming urge, leading to exhaustion.

Caesarean Section

A caesarean section (c-section) is an operation where the baby is surgically removed by an obstetrician, through an incision made in the woman's abdomen and another through the wall of the uterus. Having attended many c-sections, I can honestly say that this can be a lovely, calm and reasonably relaxed way for a baby to be born. In some cases, performing a c-section can be life saving, and we are very lucky to have this relatively safe alternative option for childbirth, in the event that the mother or baby need help. It is still important to remember, however, that a c-section is major abdominal surgery, and comes with a list of typical side effects that should be considered, including: chance of infection, excessive bleeding, development of a blood clot, damage to the bladder and breathing difficulties for the baby. In addition, both mother and baby can develop gut health issues caused by the use of antibiotics pre-and post-surgery.

Three Types of Caesarean Section

Elective. This type is planned in advance, and the woman will be aware of why it is recommended by her doctor. In some instances, the mother requests a c-section and has to convince her caregivers that she is a suitable candidate. In some cases, she may have to transfer to a different doctor to achieve this request.

Emergency. This decision is made on the day of the birth and can be recommended when the mother or baby are believed to be in difficulty but their lives are not immediately threatened. It can take up to 40 minutes or more to prepare for an emergency c-section where there is no imminent danger.

Crash. Where there is an immediate life and death situation, the woman is put to sleep so the baby can be born quickly. In this instance, you will not be permitted to attend the birth.

Rising Rates of C-Sections

In the 1950s, at the point where most births moved from home to hospital, only 3% of births in England were by c-section. By the early 1980s this had risen to 10%, and, in the 1990s, rates started to climb rapidly—from 12% in 1990 to 21% in 2001. A study done in October 2001 by the Royal Colleges and the National Childbirth Trust (NCT) listed the increase as being caused by:

- Lack of one-on-one care during labour, as some midwives are responsible for three women at a time
- Delivery of pre term infants
- Avoidance of litigation
- Lack of staff on maternity wards
- Maternal request
- Increased medicalisation of childbirth

- A greater number of older mothers
- Increased induction rates and obstetricians' preferences in their practices
- Multiple pregnancies due to IVF and other fertility treatments
- Medical indications for a c-section

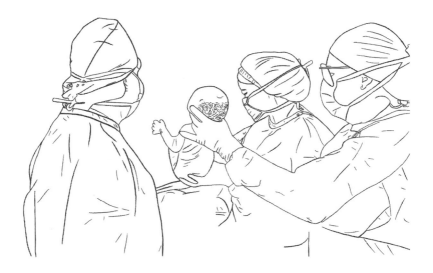

Midwife Sara Wickham talks of two additional factors to the list above that increase the risk for a c-section, which I find particularly interesting.

1. Arriving at the hospital too early in labour.

2. The mother's BMI (body mass index).

For women with a high BMI, she feels that many practitioners make assumptions based on their size, which puts them at a disadvantage. In her article 'Birth Outcomes and Women of Size', she shares the findings of a research study from Copenhagen in 2017 that said: "We found that obese women were granted fewer hours of active labour before a caesarean was performed, compared with women of normal weight." In my experience, similar issues are also faced by women who come from other minority groups. Sara Wickham describes this as 'pre-existing perceptions of the practitioner'. It is therefore important, as the birth partner, to be aware of this extra prejudice if it applies to the woman you are supporting. Be sure to ask appropriate questions if you think that:

- interventions are being offered too early, or
- she has a concern that is not being taken seriously by her doctor or midwife.

If C-Section Becomes a Reality

In the UK currently, approximately 25–35% of women will give birth via c-section. Rates vary depending on the hospital they choose to give birth in. These numbers cannot be justified as beneficial for either mother or child, and they are most likely caused by the rising rates of intervention, including induction. I assume that if you are reading this book, the woman you are supporting began her journey through pregnancy believing that she would be having a vaginal birth, so any c-section performed wouldn't have been her first choice but became her Plan B. If this is true, you might find that the recovery is difficult for her as she deals with the emotional disappointment as well as the physical healing that will take place over the months that follow.

During surgery, you can expect that there will be a large number of people in the operating theatre with you both, including a midwife, an obstetrician, the obstetrician's assistant, a theatre nurse, an anaesthetist with an assistant, and possibly a paediatrician to look after the baby. In some cases there may also be a student and if required, an interpreter. The operation is usually performed under either a spinal or epidural anaesthetic, depending on whether it is an elective or emergency c-section and whether the woman already has an effective epidural in place. Birth partners are typically shown where to change into scrubs whilst the woman is wheeled into theatre on the bed and transferred to the operating table. In most cases you will be expected to wait outside the operating theatre while the woman is prepped for surgery. You will be invited in at a point just before the procedure begins. You will be placed on a stool right next to her head and behind a draped off area, where they have prepared a sterile field. You won't be able to see much, so just hold her hand and keep her as calm and relaxed as possible. If the woman has requested skin to skin in theatre, the baby will be given to her and placed on her chest. If not, then the baby will be passed to you to hold while the doctors complete the surgery. You may also be sent into the recovery room with the baby while they finish up in theatre. They will bring the woman in on a bed shortly afterwards. This time in recovery is very precious, and, assuming the woman is feeling strong enough, encourage her to have the baby skin to skin if possible (not all women will feel ready for this; if you are a spouse or relative, you can have the baby skin to skin with you). In some instances, the baby will be taken to the special care baby unit (SCBU) for what might be a short period of time or a few days/weeks depending on the circumstances. Very rarely the baby may need to be transferred to another hospital, depending on the severity of the baby's condition or the space available in the SCBU of the hospital you are in.

IMPORTANT TO KNOW   *Typically all your bags and belongings will have been taken to recovery at the time of the c-section, so you will not be going back to the room you had previously occupied and will most likely go straight to the postnatal ward. You can ask if there is a private room available, as some hospitals will save these for women who experience a more complicated birth, giving them privacy while they recover.*

Death of a Baby

Although this is a difficult subject to cover, I think it is important to acknowledge that sometimes, sadly, a baby may die during pregnancy, birth or the early postnatal period. Whilst rare, if this does happen to the woman you are supporting, you both have my deepest sympathy. Usually a specialist bereavement midwife is on hand to help families experiencing baby loss, as there are some difficult decisions to be made at this time. For example, if labour hasn't already started, the woman will need to decide if she should wait for it to begin on its own or if an induction or c-section are preferable based on her individual circumstances. In this instance, recognise that she will hold the memories of this birth dear to her for the rest of her life, and so her experience of birth even in the midst of grief and shock still matters. No one who provides care for her should assume what her preferences are, and she should be able to achieve whatever elements of her birth plan she wants to. This is still her body and this is an experience that is happening to her—she is not merely a vessel. Facilities may vary at each hospital, and once the baby is born, the bereavement midwife should help you discover what options are available to care for the baby before saying goodbye. This may include having the baby stay with the parents in a special cold cot, and having the opportunity to organise a memory box, photos, or hand and foot prints.

QUICK RECAP

Here are the main things to remember when discussing Plan B.

- **During pregnancy.** If a complication arises during pregnancy, for either the woman or the baby, she may need to consider Plan B. This can be upsetting, but at least it will give her some time to look at other options and discuss them in detail with you and her care providers.
- **What are her risk factors?** Look in detail at her particular risk factors and try to ensure she is not just 'ticking a box' and ending up with an intervention when in fact it doesn't necessarily apply to her.
- **What are tests for?** Ensure that she understands what all tests offered to her are for, what the implications of the results will mean to her, and any other relevant information before accepting or declining.

- **What is her Bishop's Score?** If an induction is offered, she can ask the midwife for her Bishop's Score. This will give her the chance to have an informed discussion with her midwife and doctor about her options.
- **Positions for Plan B.** Consider labour positions for Plan B, so in the event that she is only able to use a bed, she knows how to maximise the room she has in her pelvis.
- **Preferences for Plan B.** In case Plan B becomes necessary during labour, talk to her about how she feels regarding the use of forceps, ventouse or c-section during a birth planning session. Ask her to clarify her preferences should any of these become a reality.

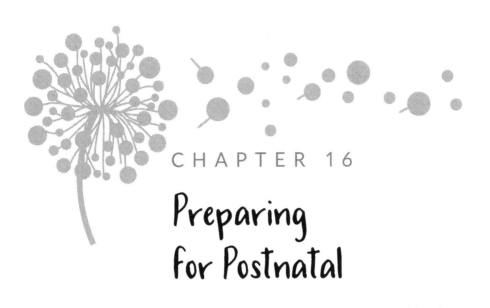

CHAPTER 16

Preparing for Postnatal

She found when she mothered her own way, she mothered her best way.

–January Harshe

Note: Throughout this chapter I refer to the baby as he, and the mother as she.

The early seconds, minutes and hours of a newborn baby's life are extremely important and quite fundamental to the bonding process, the feeding process and the seeding process. Just like any other mammal on this planet, the young human depends on its mother for survival, and we have only recently begun to realise that this is a sacred time that we should not rush. The immediate need of the baby is to be kept warm, so the mother's body steps up and becomes a human incubator. Her temperature will rise if the baby is cold, and cool down if the baby is hot. During the golden hour (see Chapter 7), if the mother and baby are left untouched as one unit for as long as possible, an abundance of hormones are released. She will produce high levels of oxytocin—which are required for the placenta to separate from the uterine wall— and her prolactin levels will also start to rise. This process is essential for bonding and breastfeeding. As the baby continues to lay on his mother's chest or abdomen, his breathing and temperature begins to stabilise, and his body is exposed to his mother's bacteria, which colonises his gut.

Newborn Checks

When the baby is first born, the midwife will be observing the baby and recording how he looks at birth. An Apgar score (visual score to assess a newborn's health) is taken at one minute and again at five minutes old. The midwife is looking to check the baby's heart rate, breathing, colour, tone and reflexes, and a low score could indicate that the baby needs help. When the mother and baby have had some skin-to-skin time, ideally at least an hour, the midwife will ask to weigh the baby. At this point they may also measure his head circumference, which will then be recorded in the baby's health record. Before the baby goes home, he will have a full newborn check called a NIPE (Newborn and Infant Physical Examination). This involves checking the baby over from head to toe: hips, eyes, mouth, heart, and, if male, his testes. The baby will also be offered a hearing test shortly after birth. Some babies may be required to remain in hospital for up to 24 or 48 hours to have extra observations depending on risk factors during pregnancy, or if an issue arose during labour or birth. If a risk of infection was suspected, it can be longer, as the paediatricians may need to wait for test results to come back. During this time the mother and/or baby may be offered intravenous antibiotics every 12 hours as a precaution.

SCBU

In the event that the baby is born and is a little slow to breathe, you will usually notice the midwife rub the baby. This is perfectly normal, and many babies take time to transition as their lungs inflate. As the umbilical cord remains attached, the baby will still be receiving oxygen. If the baby continues to struggle, the midwife may ask you as the birth partner to press the buzzer to call for help if there is no one else in the room. In the event that the baby needs extra support to breathe or if there is another medical issue, the midwife or paediatrician present may feel it is best to remove the baby from the umbilical cord and take him across to a designated space that is set aside for resuscitation. If the baby doesn't make a quick recovery, he may be taken to the Special Care Baby Unit (SCBU) for further support and observation. As the birth partner, depending on if you are a spouse or relative, you might be able to go with the baby. In some families, this is the preference rather than you remaining with the mother, and you should discuss this in pregnancy. If the mother has been sleeping with a few muslin cloths or blankets, (see Chapter 7) you can take them with you at this time to give the baby as much chance as possible to be colonised by the family's bacteria. In most cases the trip to SCBU is precautionary and the baby comes back to the mother very quickly. Always ask any doctors involved to explain what they are doing to the baby, and remember that if you are one of the parents, you should still have a say in the treatment of your child and reasonable discussions should take place with the paediatrician where possible. Once in SCBU, the staff are usually very proactive in helping the parents provide as much of the care as possible. If the mother would like to breastfeed, she can be helped to express colostrum and milk which can be given to the baby through a tube if he is unable to be with her.

Vitamin K

In the immediate period after the birth (usually within an hour or two) the midwife will ask the woman and her partner if they would like the baby to have Vitamin K. This can be given via an injection in one dose, orally in three doses, or the parents can decline. The routine 'offer' of Vitamin K is to prevent a condition known as Vitamin K Deficiency Bleeding (VKDB). Whilst it is rare, it is considered unpredictable, so the decision was made in the 1940s for all babies to be given Vitamin K as a preventative measure to help their blood to clot. I have provided some links to interesting articles on Vitamin K in the Resources section on my website so that you can both find out more about the options, ensuring a well informed decision can be made in advance of the birth.

Bottle Feeding

If a mother knows from the outset that she would like to bottle feed, it is important to acknowledge that decision is best for both her and the baby. There is a lot of information available online about what she will need to purchase, including the bottles and sterilising equipment. She can speak to her midwife about what formula milk is recommended and suitable for a newborn. It is very important that the mother doesn't forget the benefits of skin-to-skin, which are not just for breastfed babies— all babies, regardless of how they are fed, can be held close to their mothers. Those precious newborn snuggles will deepen their bond as the baby adjusts to life outside the womb.

Breastfeeding

If the woman you are supporting decides to breastfeed, then it is important for her to be fully aware of the pros and cons, so that she understands the level of commitment involved from the outset. This is not meant to put her off, but help her to prepare for the correct level of physical and emotional assistance she may require. In my experience, if a woman is not well cared for through the process of learning how to breastfeed, she can flounder and give up. In the Resources section at the back there are links to websites that will provide more detailed information about breastfeeding that will support any woman and her partner through the journey.

The Breast Crawl

If a newborn baby is left on his mother's abdomen, he has the instinctive ability to slowly crawl upwards and attach to the breast. There are many steps to the process, and it takes great patience to give the baby the space and time to achieve this. If the woman you are supporting would like her baby to have the opportunity to self-latch, it is essential that you both recognise this time be unhurried. During his efforts of maneuvering himself closer to the nipple you may notice him smelling his hands, using his feet to push himself up his mother's body, and moving his head and neck to edge himself closer. He will be very alert at times, and may sleep in between movements. Try not to touch or help him to reach his destination, because this will undo his hard work and he will have to go back to step one. If at any point in those first few hours, a well-meaning midwife offers to help by suggesting 'let's see if we can get this baby latched on for a feed', the woman should not feel under pressure to accept. Sometimes this can be encouraged too early when the baby is not ready. In this instance the comment 'not right now' should be enough to say no, thank you, and the mother can carry on with keeping the baby skin to skin and remaining relaxed.

Milk Production

During pregnancy and the early days of a baby's life, milk supply is hormone driven. A woman begins producing colostrum (baby's first milk) as early as the second trimester, and it is ready and available for the baby to access as soon as he is born. It is thick, sticky and very concentrated. The baby has to work hard to obtain a few drops, which is all he needs initially to sustain energy in those early hours and days. This is because his newborn tummy is so tiny.

Described as liquid gold, colostrum:

- Helps build your baby's immune system with antibodies, providing protection.
- Helps line the gut and encourages the growth of good bacteria.
- Provides the baby with proteins, antioxidants and other key nutrients.
- Regulates the body and helps adjust to life outside the womb.
- Acts as a natural laxative, clearing out unneeded waste.

As progesterone lowers and prolactin levels rise, the body begins to produce milk, which tends to 'come in' typically around three days after birth, but in some cases can be on day two, four or five. A woman's breasts make milk on a supply and demand basis. Milk doesn't just sit around as if it was in a warehouse going out of date. Breasts are factories, and they produce to the level of demand that the baby orders. This means that as the baby feeds, the body registers how much milk to make tomorrow. Milk is being produced all the time, with the speed of production determined by how completely the baby empties the breast. The website **kellymom.com** calls it a 'use it or lose it' production. No demand = no supply. In order to succeed, the baby will need to latch well and feed effectively, making sure to get as much of the areola in the mouth as possible, and not sucking on just the nipple. At the same time as the baby receives all his nutrients from his mother, he will also begin to receive his antibodies, which are made specifically for each baby's requirements and passed through via the breastmilk.

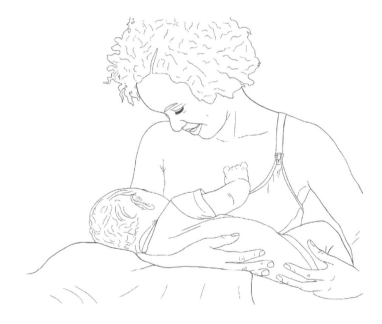

Breastfeeding Checklist for Birth Partners

Here are my top tips for the first 24 hours.

- The baby has had plenty of nourishment in the womb before birth, so he may not be hungry initially. If the baby doesn't look interested in feeding, just keep him skin to skin where possible.

- The baby should have his tummy held in close to the mother's body. The mother should keep her fingers away from her nipples, and the nipple should line up with the baby's nose.
- The baby should take a wide mouthful of the mother's areola around the nipple and not suck on the nipple itself.
- The mother can try rubbing her nipple on the baby's top lip to encourage the baby to open his mouth wide.
- Ideally the baby will have his first feed within six hours of being born.
- If after six hours the baby hasn't fed, the mother can hand express a few drops of colostrum to help the baby lick the drops.
- A baby only needs approximately three feeds in the first 24 hours.
- If the baby hasn't fed within 12 hours, continue to hand express colostrum and give it to the baby every two to three hours. This can be fed to the baby via a cup or syringe, so ask the midwife for help.
- Alternative positions may be tried by the mother, such as lying down on her side with the baby lying beside her. This can help because she no longer has to hold the baby, and she may feel more relaxed.
- If the mother is receiving conflicting advice from well meaning midwives or maternity support workers, my advice, where possible, is to go home and get professional help! By engaging with a properly trained breastfeeding councillor, she will receive consistent support and feel confident that the person she is speaking to is incredibly well trained. I recommend she find out what support is available locally during the pregnancy, and have all telephone numbers and information in her notes so you can find them easily. The majority of support is free through the NHS or volunteer helpline numbers. In some cases there may be a small charge for one-to-one support in her own home.
- It is important that the mother is not too stressed when trying to feed. Encourage her to relax her shoulders, soften her jaw and breathe. The less tense she is, the easier it will be for the baby to latch.

- By day two, the baby will begin feeding more frequently, and the feeds will ramp up to 8-12 feeds in every 24 hour period. At least two of these feeds should be at night.

IMPORTANT TO KNOW *Beware that night two is usually one where the baby cries all night. It's common enough to have a name—'second night syndrome'. It is thought that having slept off the birth, the baby is beginning to adjust to his new surroundings, working hard to build up his mother's milk supply.*

> If breastfeeding is not going well in hospital, get home and get help!

Breastfeeding Pros and Cons

I guess the biggest pro to breastfeeding is to state the obvious, starting with the old slogan 'human milk for human babies'. A woman's body is made to breastfeed her young. The food she produces contains exactly the right nutrients that her baby needs to grow and develop. It is served at exactly the right temperature for the baby, it is easy to access, and no sterilisation is required. It is both food and water, and if it's a hot day, the water content in the milk will be exactly what the baby needs to quench its thirst. Likewise, when the baby is having a growth spurt, he can feed for long periods of time, accessing higher fat milk and increasing the supply. Choosing to breastfeed is a big commitment that takes time; a mother will also need to eat healthily and reduce caffeine and alcohol levels. In the early weeks, a woman may feel trapped and believe that feeding the baby is all she does, which can, for some women, lead to difficulty bonding with her baby. It can be a messy business with leaks and stains, and in some cases it can also be painful, with cracked nipples, engorgement and mastitis being three of the most common issues that can occur. Pain is usually the result of the way the baby is latching on to the breast. It could also be a sign that the baby has a tongue tie—a condition where the strip of skin connecting the baby's tongue to the bottom of his mouth is shorter than usual. This can restrict the movement of the tongue, which can make it harder for some babies to breastfeed. Both of these problems can be resolved quickly with help from a specialist, who can suggest alternative positions and attachment advice, and might also recommend a simple procedure called tongue-tie division.

Signs of a Tongue Tie

- A baby that can do "the crawl" but can't attach at the end.
- A baby that 'bobs' a lot then gives up.
- A baby who feeds ALL the time and doesn't gain weight.
- A baby who makes a clicking sound during feeding.
- A nipple that is misshapen or "white" at the tip after feeding.
- A baby that seems very windy.
- A baby that dribbles whilst feeding.
- Often babies with a tongue tie are mistakenly diagnosed as having 'reflux'.

Deciding to Stop Breastfeeding

If, for whatever reason the mother has decided to move on from breastfeeding, then she should be helped to do so, no questions asked. If, however, her supply is diminishing and she needs help before she decides what she really wants to do, then encourage her to seek support before it is too late. Check in with her, so you know that if she does decide to stop, she will never regret the decision, because just like the marathon analogy in Chapter 3, she could be devastated if it turns out she quit because she felt unsupported. It is resentments like these that can affect her for years to come. Try looking into the following reasons she is considering stopping.

- If breastfeeding is making her sore and upset, help her to speak to a professional breastfeeding councillor to identify if there are any easy ways to correct her or the baby's position.

- Triple check that the baby does not have a tongue tie that is causing issues and was missed by the midwife.

- Make sure she is not feeling under pressure from her partner or other family members to stop feeding; they may not understand how deep seated her feelings are about breastfeeding.

- Sometimes the other parent wants more of a role with the baby and would like to be involved in feeding, so learning how to express milk—a few weeks after birth—can solve this problem.

SAM'S STORY Sam had attended an antenatal course with five other couples. They all had varying birth experiences, and the early postnatal period was a time that they shared messages but hadn't managed to meet up. When the babies were around eight weeks old, all the mums came to my baby massage class and were able to see each other and talk in detail about their experiences. Sam discovered that she was the only one who was no longer breastfeeding, and she began to cry. She shared with us that she stopped feeding her baby at two weeks old. She had decided to switch to bottle feeding, and she felt at the time that it was the right decision for her as she was not enjoying her baby. She had not anticipated that the others in the group would speak of how hard their breastfeeding journeys were too, and she started to wonder if she could have continued. Despite my support and lots of reassurance from her friends, she couldn't let go of the judgement she placed on herself, and after two weeks, she decided to stop coming to the group as it was too painful for her to watch the other mums feed their babies.

Sam's story is a recent one, and one I don't share lightly. It is unfortunately typical of many that I have witnessed over the years. In my experience, no one judges a woman for her feeding choice more than the woman herself. If I work with a client who is deciding to end her breastfeeding journey, I encourage her to hold her head high and be proud to share that she knows that a happy mum equals a happy baby. No one else is living inside her body or her brain, so she must let go of any self-doubt or self-judgement. As long as she is making a well informed decision, and not making the decision based on the fact that she is exhausted and sore, then she can always feel confident that she is stopping for the right reasons! Education and preparation before birth can help every woman understand the difficult hurdles breastfeeding sometimes presents, so she will be well prepared to get help if she needs it. I have shared some excellent breastfeeding resources at the back of the book.

> A baby in the womb is held on demand and fed on demand.

The Fourth Trimester

Dr Harvey Karp, an American paediatrician, coined the phrase 'the fourth trimester' when he spoke of the first 3 months of life, where a baby simply wants to be held all the time in a womb-like environment. He speaks of the womb as the most wonderful space for a baby. It is not only lovely and warm, but he is held in a cradled, comfortable position, listening to the sound of his mother's voice and her heart beating in her chest. The baby can eat whenever he wants, and he is rocked to sleep as his mum goes about her day. All needs are met—all of the time. It is the most perfect place to be. During those first 12 weeks of life, knowing and understanding that the baby will want to be permanently held in their arms can make it easier for new parents. Even when exhausted, being prepared will help them to recognise that the baby is transitioning, and the need to be so close to a parent's body won't last forever.

Using a Sling

As the baby is most comfortable feeling safe, warm and snug, a good quality sling is essential for the fourth trimester and beyond. It gives the baby the opportunity to be carried around, while the wearer has her or his hands free to deal with other aspects of life. I have to admit that I am particularly keen to recommend 'wrap slings' (a long piece of fabric that wraps around your body) to my clients, as they are suitable to wear from birth onwards. They hold the baby snuggly to the body and they give the baby the feeling of being back in the womb. In my experience, a well worn sling—meaning the baby is in the correct position inside—ensures that the baby sleeps well and has all its needs met for most of the day. A baby can even be fed in a sling. There are many brands out there, with lots of fancy fabrics and great colours and patterns. She and the baby will love being close to each other. The sling can also be worn by the other parent, and anyone else that is helping to care for the baby.

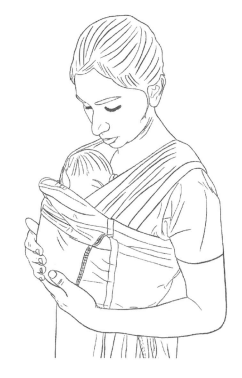

The Baby Blues

In the days following the baby's birth, the woman's hormone levels will fluctuate and her milk will come in. She should be prepared that around three to five days post birth, she may feel emotional and cry over happiness, sadness, anxiety, overwhelm—anything, to be honest—and she will not be able to explain why she is crying. Symptoms will pass, usually within a few days, but it can affect some women for a few weeks. The baby blues are harmless and normal and there is no treatment; it's just part of the journey of the early postnatal period. In the meantime, if you live with her or spend time with her regularly, try to be a stable, positive presence. Take the baby and let her sleep or read; help her with household duties; cook her a special dinner. If the symptoms linger or become worse where she appears confused, withdrawn or even 'manic' (where she is doing everything at high speed) then it could be a sign of something more serious, and you should contact the midwife or arrange an appointment with the GP.

Postnatal Depression (PND)

As time progresses and the baby grows, some women don't bounce back in the way that is considered normal. PND is something that is widely known about and feared by women and their partners. It is fair to say that because no one can truly pinpoint a cause, it seems very random as to who suffers and who doesn't. According to the Royal College of Psychiatrists, PND can affect approximately 10% of women.

The reason it can be hard to detect is because its symptoms mimic the kind of symptoms you would expect any new mum to feel—tiredness, irritability, sleeplessness, anxiety. Symptoms may go on to include avoiding others, appetite changes, an inability to enjoy anything, negative and guilty thoughts, and feelings of hopelessness. Some women have thoughts of suicide. Most women with PND do not enjoy all aspects of being a mother, but that doesn't mean that they don't love their babies. Some women describe that they don't feel that they are doing well as a mother, and are letting their baby down; this is a symptom of depression, and the woman should see a doctor.

During my antenatal courses I ask couples to consider how they can attempt to avoid PND. I encourage them to take care of these three elements.

* Good nutrition
* Good sleep
* Gut health

Good nutrition is vital during the first few months with a new baby. It is common for a new mum who is alone at home all day to skip meals or eat junk. This happens because, first, she is too tired and occupied with the baby to have time or energy to prepare food, and second, when you eat junk food, your body craves more of it. A poor diet is commonly linked to mental health conditions, and PND is no different. Menu planning in advance can help to ensure that each night she has healthy food available to eat the next day. Lack of sleep is a tough issue when a new baby is around. It is common for most women to be exhausted, and when they are overtired, it becomes even harder to sleep. Their loved ones should encourage them to catch up on sleep whenever they can, and make it a priority. Finally, I notice that women who have been exposed to antibiotics, either in pregnancy, during labour or after the birth, can experience many side effects when all the friendly bacteria in the gut is also wiped out. It is widely documented that there is a direct link between the brain and the gut, and the depletion of these protective microbes leaves the immune defenses low. Some of the most common symptoms I see in new mothers include: depression, thrush (yeast infection), skin conditions like acne and eczema, constipation and an inability to fall asleep. As the antibiotics can pass through to the baby in the womb and in breast milk, many of these symptoms occur for them too, including colic and general digestive issues. A good course of probiotics to help replenish the friendly bacteria, along with a nutritious diet, will support the gut and help to avoid the dreaded PND.

Birth Trauma

Birth trauma is a shortened phrase for someone who is suffering from post-traumatic stress disorder (PTSD). Elements of a traumatic birth could include: a long labour, a short but very painful labour, feelings of loss of control, feeling unsupported by staff, and fear of death or permanent damage. It can occur due to the birth being induced; having an instrumental birth (ventouse and/or forceps); having an emergency or crash c-section; experiencing poor pain relief or having pain relief withdrawn; or experiencing a problem with the baby, perhaps resulting in the fear that the baby would die or be taken to SCBU.

What is PTSD Following Childbirth?

It is important to understand that PTSD (Post-Traumatic Stress Disorder) is a normal set of reactions to a traumatic, scary or bad experience, and the symptoms of PTSD linked to birth include:

- Reliving the birth or parts of the birth
- Difficulty remembering parts of the birth
- Numbed emotions
- Problems bonding with the baby
- Depression, irritability or mood swings
- Difficulty concentrating
- Problems with breastfeeding
- Feelings of inadequacy
- Fear that previous events will recur with similar, if not worse, outcomes
- Fear of becoming pregnant again

Isn't This Postnatal Depression?

PTSD can overlap with postnatal depression (PND) as some of the symptoms are the same, but the two illnesses are distinct and need to be treated individually. PTSD can be experienced by the mother, birth partner or both.

It is important to talk about your experiences if this or a previous birth was traumatic in any way. Seek support from the birth listening service at the hospital where the woman you are supporting gave birth, or request a copy of her notes. She can book a private post-birth discussion session with a doula or an independent midwife who offers this service. It can be held at any point afterwards, even if many years have gone by—there is no limit.

Safe Sleeping

It is widely recommended that all babies should sleep in the same room as their parents for the first six months. It is also recommended that they should sleep on their backs, and that they should sleep separately in a cot or crib. In some cases, lack of sleep means that parents will decide to co-sleep with their baby, even if they had originally decided that having a baby in their bed was a 'no-go'. The Lullaby Trust has produced great guidelines about safe sleeping, regardless of where or how you all sleep. Their advice includes keeping the area where the baby sleeps clear of anything other than the blanket used to keep them warm, making sure that no one shares a bed with a baby if they have been drinking alcohol, smoking, or taking medication, and to avoid bed sharing if your baby was premature. You can find out more on the website at **lullabytrust.org.uk**.

IMPORTANT TO KNOW *Do not fall asleep with a baby whilst on the sofa. This is dangerous, as a baby can accidentally slip down between the cushions and suffocate.*

Nappy Changing

Expect a newborn baby to use a lot of nappies in the early weeks, as parents find their feet with changing them. The list that follows is a rough guide.

- **On Day 1:** Expect thick black poo called meconium and one or two wet nappies.
- **On Day 3:** Expect the poo to be green and the baby to be increasing in wet nappies.

- **By Day 5:** Expect the poo to be yellowish with at least three poos and five wet nappies per day.

The Postnatal Body

In the immediate hours after birth, the mother's blood loss will be assessed, and if she has had any stitches, they will either be monitored during a prolonged hospital stay, or the community midwife will check them when the mother and baby go home. During the early months with a newborn, a woman's body is healing and adapting, and whilst her hormone levels are high, it should be expected that she may be a bit 'all over the place' emotionally. As her body begins to return to normal, and her hormone levels recalibrate, she also begins to lose the excess hair that she grew during pregnancy, her skin pigmentation changes (which may be more noticeable in black and brown women), and her tummy muscles—which had separated during the pregnancy—will need support in coming back together. I know a lot of wonderful people who have written specialist books on the postnatal period; in particular look for Sophie Messager's book *Why Postnatal Recovery Matters*. Encourage the woman you are supporting to read about the importance of taking time to recover and recuperate—to nourish herself and learn how to discover her new self.

Diastasis Recti

Our abdominal muscles provide an internal corset protecting our vital organs and offering support to our spine and pelvis. They are made up of different layers of muscle: the rectus abdominis, internal and external obliques and transversus abdominis. During pregnancy, it is normal for the rectus abdominis (six-pack muscle) to begin to open to create space as the baby grows. In some cases, the tissue that connects the abdominals, the linea alba, thins or separates. It can be strained under too much pressure, and rather than the rectus abdominis muscles stretching, the linea alba overstretches or in some cases tears. This is known as a diastasis (or separation) of the rectus abdominis. In the postnatal period, the woman is left with a gap between the muscles which can take time to heal.

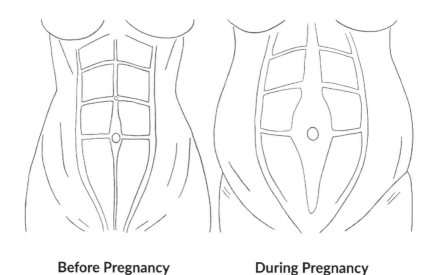

Before Pregnancy   **During Pregnancy**

Approximately two out of three women will experience long term issues caused by the separation that can lead to:

- Bladder leakage
- Weak pelvic floor muscles
- Constipation
- Lower back pain
- Poor posture

Being aware that separation of the abdominal muscles exists is essential, so that the woman does not harm herself or make the diastasis worse. Many women return to exercise too early, which can exacerbate the issue and lead to a hernia or prolapse. Encourage the woman you are supporting to make a note in her diary to seek help from a specialist nearby who has expertise in this area. I also recommend that women see a body specialist, such as a Bowen therapist, chiropractor or osteopath, no sooner than six to eight months after the baby is born to be realigned. It is important to wait, so that her hormones have a chance to diminish, but ideally not to leave it too long, as the woman should aim to be re-aligned before she becomes pregnant again. This will help to ensure good pelvic health for her in the future, and will help avoid issues like Pelvic Girdle Pain (PGP).

Resuming Sex

Many new mothers feel very unsexy in the early weeks and months after giving birth. Her body needs time to reclaim itself, her major organs are slowly moving, her muscles are shifting back together and her vagina—well, that is beginning to recover slowly too. Everything heals, the body is amazing, and all will be well soon enough. During the postnatal period, most women will share that they are exhausted. They are so tired, and they cannot imagine having the added responsibility of satisfying their partners' physical needs as well as their babies'. They may feel incredibly 'touched out' and not able to imagine what having sex again will feel like for them, let alone what would they do with the baby, as it doesn't leave their sight in those early months. What typically happens is that even though they want to be physical with their partner, they worry that a hug or a cuddle will lead the partner to think that sex is on the cards. Whether you are a spouse or not, I would open up the discussion and see what she shares with you. In my experience, once she knows that she can enjoy physical affection with her partner without it leading to sex, she will relax and begin to enjoy that side of her relationship once more.

Postnatal Doulas

Postnatal doulas, just like birth doulas, provide practical, emotional, physical and informational support to new parents. Their role is to ensure that those early days go as smoothly as possible and that the family members are nurtured and cared for as they navigate through life with a newborn. The concept has been around for thousands of years, with local women caring for the new mother during those early postnatal weeks so that she can recover from birth and learn how to take care of the baby. In the absence of help from family or friends, hiring a postnatal doula can be a really good option. The doula, who builds a trusting relationship with the mother, can help with instruction on caring for the baby, feeding support, emotional support, practical support with household management, preparing meals, or helping the mother rest or have a bath. In my case, I have also taken a client shopping for feeding bras, helped bath the baby, bought basic shopping items, collected older children from school, helped with the ironing and much more. Typically families would consider hiring a postnatal doula for the first six to eight weeks, although many will carry on support for several months if required. You can find local postnatal doulas listed on the doula UK website, **doula.org.uk.**

Postnatal Plan

Just like a birth plan, every woman should write a postnatal plan before the birth to help her think about and work out what life will be like 'on the other side' of pregnancy, and what level of support she might ask from her loved ones as she navigates those early months. Consideration for this period of time is incredibly important, and to leave it off the agenda makes a couple incredibly underprepared for parenting.

There should be several sections to the plan. I recommend starting with the following.

- What do I need in the first two weeks?
- What do I need in the first three months (the adjustment period also known as the fourth trimester)?
- What do I need in the first six months?

If you are a relative, spouse, postnatal doula or other caregiver, you can sit down with her and discuss each of these sections. Ask her to think about who she would want around her—and who she might not.

The First Two Weeks

- Who will come and bring food?
- Who will clean and help out with chores?
- Who are you happy to see while you are in your underwear and trying to establish feeding?
- Who would you trust to hold your baby while you showered?
- Who would be there for your needs (not just the baby's)?
- If these people don't exist, how will you cope?
- How much does breastfeeding mean to you? Have you got the details for breastfeeding support locally? (This is vital!)

During the first two weeks, she will experience the biggest hormonal dip of her entire life so far. It will affect her emotions and her mood and she needs someone to support her through this. She is likely to cry for no reason, as she experiences the 'baby blues'. Once her milk comes in around day three or four she will also be sore and may feel like she isn't coping. This is the time for a smile, a nod of understanding, a hug, and a bar of chocolate, not well meaning advice (unless she asks for it) or a 'fix it' approach.

The First Three Months

During the 'fourth trimester', a new mother should expect to get very little done, as the baby will want to be held practically all of the time. It is important to try to surrender to that, not resist it. As her support network begins to reduce their help, perhaps when they go back to work and the woman is home alone all day with the baby, she should consider what options she has locally to help her. She can practice asking for help during pregnancy, so that it is easier for her in the early postnatal period. She should be encouraged to instigate support by saying 'I need help', or 'I need to talk'. Remind her to express her needs and desires to her partner (if that is not you), and explain how important communication is. If she resists, point out the capabilities of anyone that tries to do everything with only one arm, and encourage her to buy a really good wrap sling to hold the baby close. During pregnancy, encourage her to consider sharing her ideas about those early months with any family members who might have opinions about parenthood that do not align with her philosophies. For example: If it is important to her to have the baby with her at all times, tell her to talk about how she has researched the benefits of the baby being held a lot in those early weeks. She can send out copies of articles about the fourth trimester to well meaning grandparents, friends or relatives who may believe you can spoil a baby by holding them too much. If she thinks she may struggle with an untidy home, encourage her to consider how the lack of control might make her feel. Make a sensible plan about what she thinks could be achieved each day, rather than thinking she is failing if she doesn't manage to get anything done. Discussing and acknowledging what she might feel like during this time makes the postnatal period a lot easier. This plan can then be revisited after the baby is born and adapted or tweaked if she realises some elements are working and some are not.

The First Six Months

Her partner needs to be involved in writing this plan, and they both need to be involved in maintaining communication. The first six months of a baby's life can be a huge strain on a relationship, no matter how deep the foundations. It is useful to anticipate what the effects might be on both their lives, and how they can support each other through it—physically, mentally and financially. If the woman is breastfeeding, she is likely to be incredibly sleep deprived over a prolonged period of time. This is a commitment that takes courage and dedication, and any partner needs to maintain support and gratitude for the incredible job she is doing. She may feel murderous when she is up for the fourth time in a night, and her partner is snoring away, so it is important for them to schedule some focused time each week when they can connect and talk about anything other than the baby for an agreed period of time. If a babysitter is an option, great; if not, encourage her to use the sling, so that she can at least hold hands with her partner whilst out on a walk, for example. In addition, she needs to surround herself with a great network of people who are going to hold her and support her through the journey of early parenthood, and not bring her down or question her instincts and decisions as a mother.

QUICK RECAP

Here are the main things to remember when discussing the postnatal period.

- **Skin to skin.** The baby can stay skin to skin for hours, days, and weeks. Once families have dressed the baby after the initial 'golden hour', they often forget all about the benefits.
- **You cannot spoil a newborn baby.** Even if people tell you that you can spoil your baby by holding him all the time, this is not true. No one will make a rod for their own back by holding the baby too much. Send well meaning friends and relatives information on the fourth trimester.
- **Babies will cry.** A baby will still have bouts of crying regardless of how much you hold him, as crying is his only means of communication. Consider wearing a sling to keep him close while leaving your hands free.
- **Make a postnatal plan.** In order to ensure maximum support during the postnatal period while the woman recovers from pregnancy and birth, it is essential to make a postnatal plan.
- **Help should be appropriate in meeting her needs.** She doesn't have to hand the baby over to anyone if she doesn't want to. Others should support and care for her and the household and let her take care of the baby. The woman may need time to recover before having to cope with family members who might set her back in her postnatal recovery.

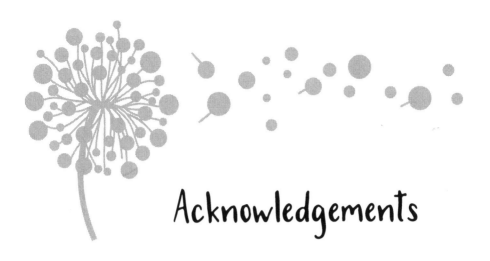

Acknowledgements

To my husband, Tim. Thank you for your unwavering support throughout the process of writing this book. For bringing me endless cups of coffee, and for reading every single page when I needed a male perspective on the content. Your belief in me spurred me on and kept me going throughout this incredible journey.

To my four wonderful children, Joe, Lauren, Caitlin and Darcy. I love being your mother and continue to enjoy every moment, watching you develop into incredible, funny, loving and kind adults. You are my inspiration for writing this book, as I hope to do my best to ensure that each one of your future children's births are magical.

To my mother, Maureen, and my father, Malcolm. Thank you both for being such incredible parents to Nick and I. For always believing in us and making our lives so special.

To Sophie Beresford and Fiona Gordon, who poured many hours into reading this book and offered me huge pearls of their wisdom. Your words flow through the chapters, and you have made it so much better than that first original draft. I am incredibly grateful to you both.

To Darcy Beresford, who patiently and expertly sketched each image, not once but twice.

To Debbie Aglietti, who inspired me to become a doula all those years ago, and who has been a huge source of support to me ever since.

To all the women and their partners who have invited me to be a part of their birth journeys. Every single one has had an impact on my life, and I feel privileged and grateful to you all.

To everyone who has given me permission to use their words in this book—you know who you are.

And finally, to Tessa Avila. Thank you so much for helping me to give birth to this baby. Not only are you my dear friend, but you have been my editor, designer and mentor throughout. You have been a constant source of humour, support, encouragement, information and patience. You breathed light into the pages and for that I will be forever grateful. I am truly blessed to have had you walk alongside me as my 'book doula', and I couldn't be more proud of what we achieved.

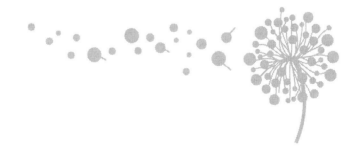

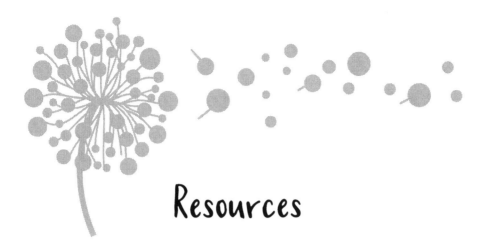

Resources

To make it easier for you to access information from these websites, I have included a copy of all the clickable links on my website, organised by chapter. From there, you will also be able to access the free downloads that accompany this book: **birthability.co.uk/links-and-resources/**

Antenatal Education

Birthability   **birthability.co.uk**

Births of Multiples

Twins Trust   **twinstrust.org**

Birth Support

Doula UK   **doula.org.uk**

Independent Midwives UK   **imuk.org.uk**

Birth Trauma

Birth Trauma Association   **birthtraumaassociation.org.uk**

Breastfeeding Support

Breastfeeding Support   **breastfeeding.support**

Kelly Mom   **kellymom.com**

Association for Breastfeeding Mothers   **abm.me.uk**

La Leche League   **laleche.org.uk**

Caesarean Birth

Caesarean Birth   **caesarean.org.uk**

Evidence-Based Resources

Mothers and Babies Reducing Risks through Audits (MBRRACE-UK)
npeu.ox.ac.uk/mbrrace-uk

Midwife Thinking   **midwifethinking.com**

Evidence Based Birth   **evidencebasedbirth.com**

Sara Wickham   **sarawickham.com**

Sarah Buckley   **sarahbuckley.com**

Freebirth

Samantha Gadsden   **caerphillydoula.co.uk**

Guidelines

Royal College of Obstetricians and Gynaecologists   **rcog.org.uk**

National Institute for Health and Care Excellence (NICE)   **nice.org.uk**

Royal College of Midwives (RCM)   **rcm.org.uk**

Royal College of Anaesthetists (RCoA)   **rcoa.ac.uk**

Royal College of Paediatrics and Child Health (RCPCH)   **rcpch.ac.uk**

Cochrane (Summaries of health evidence)   **cochrane.org**

Miscarriage and Stillbirth

Stillbirth and Neonatal Death Charity (Sands) **sands.org.uk**

Lullaby Trust **lullabytrust.org.uk**

Tommy's **tommys.org**

Beyond Bea **beyondbea.co.uk**

Optimal Cord Clamping

Wait for White Campaign waitforwhite.com

Ticc Tocc Campaign **drgreen.com**

Lotus Birth **babyprepping.com**

Placenta Encapsulation

Placenta Remedies Network (PRN) **placentaremediesnetwork.org**

Pre- and Postnatal Depression

PaNDAS (PND Awareness and Support) **pandasfoundation.org.uk**

Pregnancy

Pregnancy Sickness Support **pregnancysicknesssupport.org.uk**

Tell Me a Good Birth Story **tellmeagoodbirthstory.com**

Spinning Babies **spinningbabies.com**

Pelvic Partnership (Pelvic Girdle Pain) **pelvicpartnership.org.uk**

Pre-Eclampsia **preeclampsia.org**

Breech Birthing **breechbirthing.com**

Gloria Lemay **wisewomanwayofbirth.com**

Rebozo techniques **sophiemessager.com**

Reduced Fetal Movement

Kicks Count **kickscount.org.uk**

Support for Women's Rights in Childbirth

Association for Improvement in Maternity Services (AIMS)

aims.org.uk

Birthrights   **birthrights.org.uk**

National Maternity Voices (NMV) / Maternity Voices Partnership (MVP)

nationalmaternityvoices.org.uk

White Ribbon Alliance   **whiteribbonalliance.org**

Maternity Action   **maternityaction.org.uk**

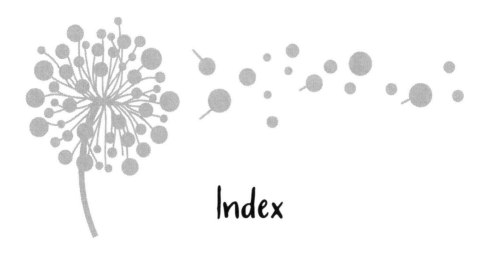

Index

A

acupressure 201
adrenaline 54–55
  ways to reduce 56
affirmations for hypnobirthing 186
Am I Allowed (AIMS) 235
amnihook 265
anchors for hypnobirthing 186
Android pelvis shape 130
Anthropoid pelvis shape 130
antibiotics
  for group B strep 259
  human microbiome and 122
  postnatal depression and 292
  premature rupture of membranes and
    73
Apgar score 280
aromatherapy 201
arriving at hospital too early 77
  as risk for caesarean section 274
  questions to ask 79
assisted birth 270
  RCOG statistics on 272
Association for Improvement in
    Maternity Services (AIMS) 13
  Am I Allowed 235
augmentation of labour
  natural methods for 267

B

baby blues
  postnatal depression vs 291
'back to back'. *See* occiput posterior (OP)
Baroness Julia Cumberlege 12

Beech, Beverley 13. *See also* Association
    for Improvement in Maternity
    Services (AIMS)
'being not doing' 167
being on call 149
  Dos and Don'ts 150
Better Births report (NHS, 2016) 12
birth bag 29, 29–30
  snack ideas for 153
birth experience
  post-birth discussions about 246–248
  taking ownership of 234–235
  trauma/PTSD and 248–249, 293
birthing pool. *See* water birth
'Birth Outcomes and Women of Size'
    (Wickham) 274
birth plans
  as a way to maintain positive control
    175
  changing 222
  checklist 213
  defined 211
  effective 218
  ineffective 217
  introducing to doctor or midwife 221
  postnatal 298–301
  questions to ask 10
Birth Skills (Sundin and Murdoch) 199
births of multiples
  high-risk pathway and 255
Bishop's score 263
bladder, importance of emptying during
    labour 156
blankets
  for use in protecting baby's microbiome
    123, 281